EASY BBQ

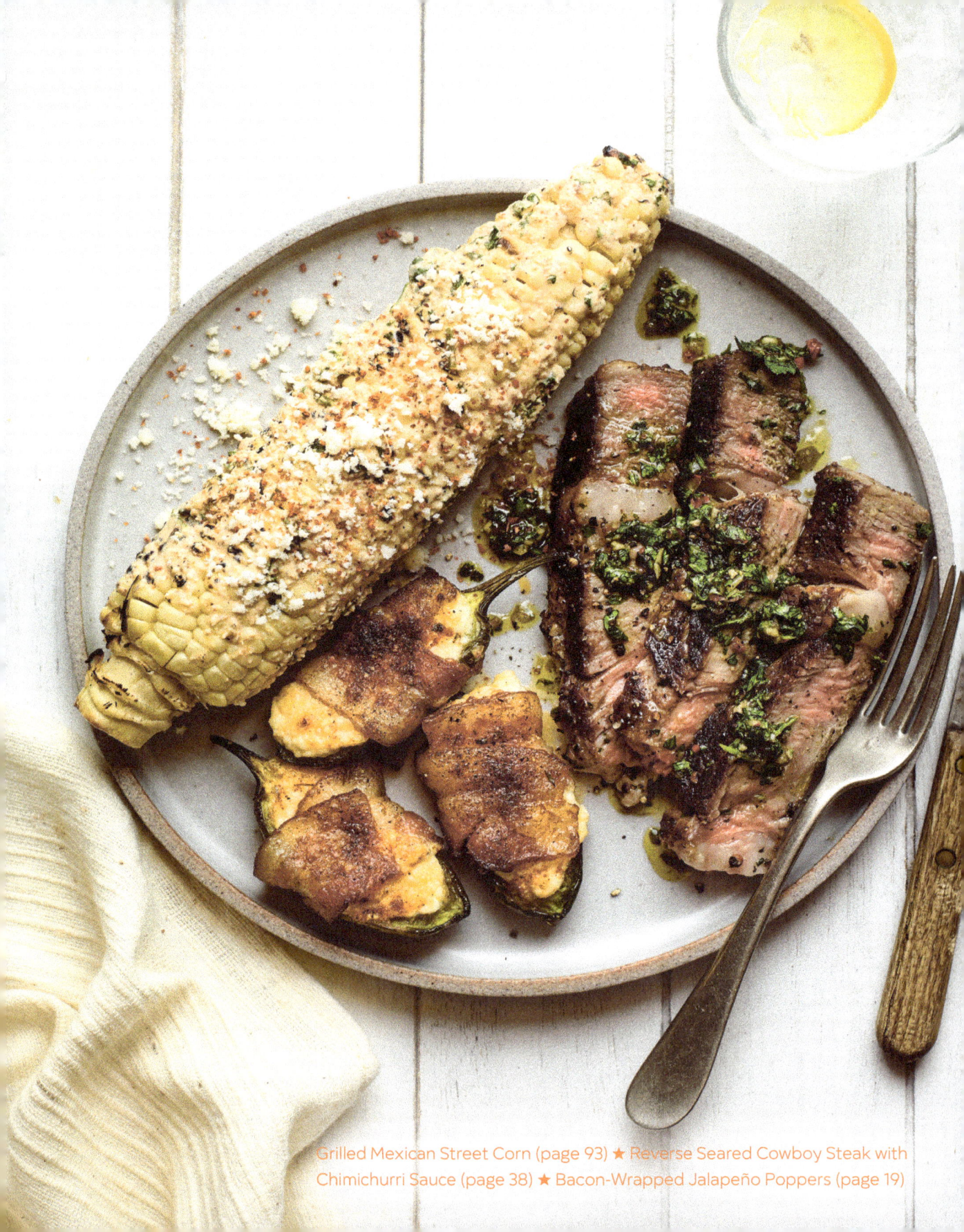

Grilled Mexican Street Corn (page 93) ★ Reverse Seared Cowboy Steak with Chimichurri Sauce (page 38) ★ Bacon-Wrapped Jalapeño Poppers (page 19)

EASY BBQ

SIMPLE, FLAVORFUL RECIPES FOR HOME GRILLING

GLENN CONNAUGHTON

Photography by Andrew Purcell

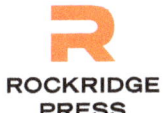

ROCKRIDGE PRESS

Copyright © 2022 by Rockridge Press, Oakland, California

No part of this publication may be reproduced, stored in a retrieval system, or transmitted in any form or by any means, electronic, mechanical, photocopying, recording, scanning, or otherwise, except as permitted under Sections 107 or 108 of the 1976 United States Copyright Act, without the prior written permission of the Publisher. Requests to the Publisher for permission should be addressed to the Permissions Department, Rockridge Press, 1955 Broadway, Suite 400, Oakland, CA 94612.

Limit of Liability/Disclaimer of Warranty: The Publisher and the author make no representations or warranties with respect to the accuracy or completeness of the contents of this work and specifically disclaim all warranties, including without limitation warranties of fitness for a particular purpose. No warranty may be created or extended by sales or promotional materials. The advice and strategies contained herein may not be suitable for every situation. This work is sold with the understanding that the Publisher is not engaged in rendering medical, legal, or other professional advice or services. If professional assistance is required, the services of a competent professional person should be sought. Neither the Publisher nor the author shall be liable for damages arising herefrom. The fact that an individual, organization, or website is referred to in this work as a citation and/or potential source of further information does not mean that the author or the Publisher endorses the information the individual, organization, or website may provide or recommendations they/it may make. Further, readers should be aware that websites listed in this work may have changed or disappeared between when this work was written and when it is read.

For general information on our other products and services or to obtain technical support, please contact our Customer Care Department within the United States at (866) 744-2665, or outside the United States at (510) 253-0500.

Rockridge Press publishes its books in a variety of electronic and print formats. Some content that appears in print may not be available in electronic books, and vice versa.

TRADEMARKS: Rockridge Press and the Rockridge Press logo are trademarks or registered trademarks of Callisto Media Inc. and/or its affiliates, in the United States and other countries, and may not be used without written permission. All other trademarks are the property of their respective owners. Rockridge Press is not associated with any product or vendor mentioned in this book.

Interior and Cover Designer: Heather Krakora
Art Producer: Hannah Dickerson
Editor: Georgia Freedman
Production Editor: Matthew Burnett
Production Manager: Holly Haydash

Photography © 2022 Andrew Purcell; food styling by Carrie Purcell. All illustrations used under license from Shutterstock.com.
Author photograph courtesy of Vida Connaughton.

Paperback ISBN: 978-1-63807-304-8
eBook ISBN: 978-1-63807-164-8
R0

To my wife and best friend, Vida, who will forever be my partner in everything we do, and to my special little angels, Kohan and Olivia, who have made being a grandpa a joyous new chapter in my life.

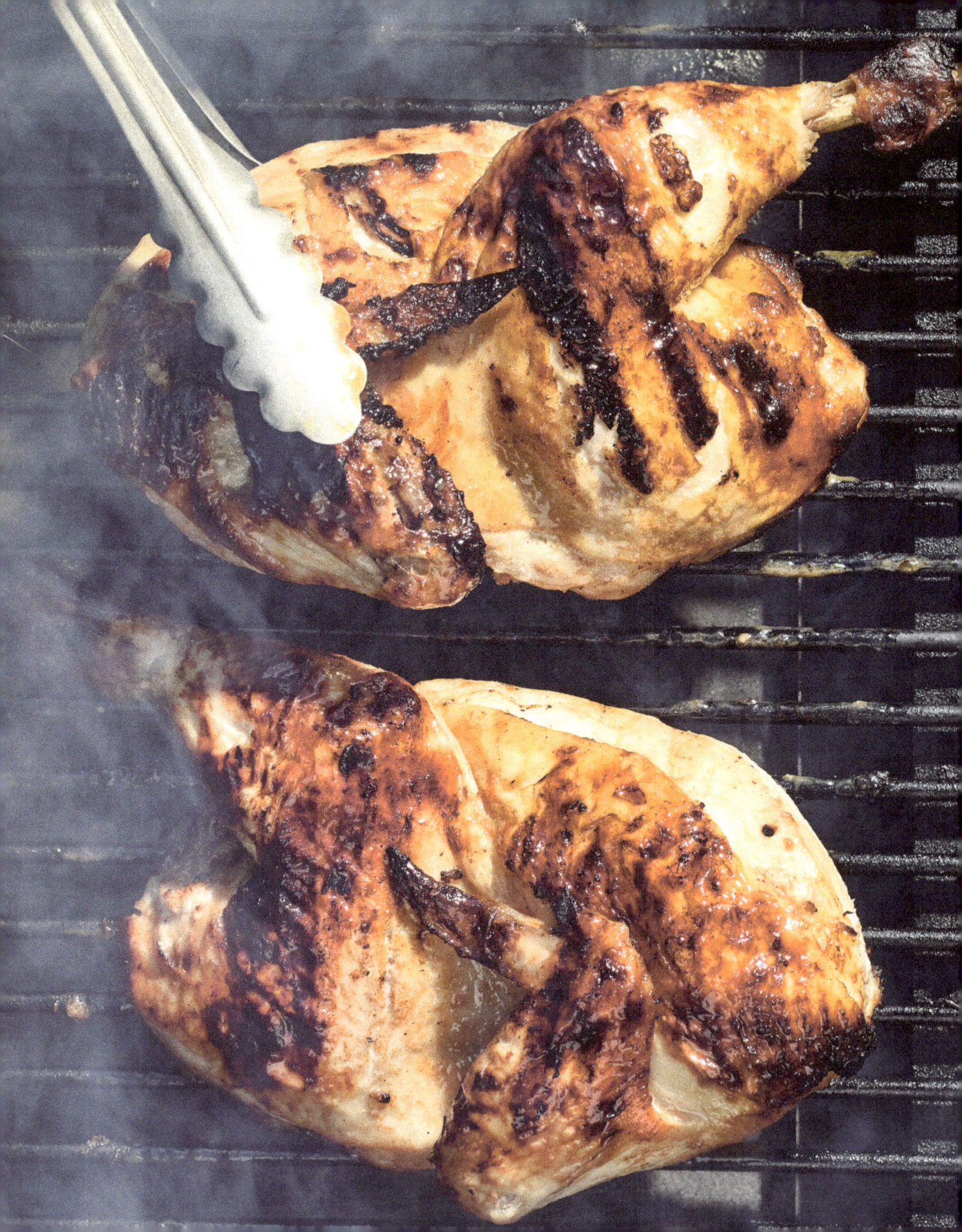

CONTENTS

INTRODUCTION **ix**

CHAPTER 1: Easy BBQ Basics 1

CHAPTER 2: Appetizers 17

CHAPTER 3: Beef and Pork 27

CHAPTER 4: Poultry 49

CHAPTER 5: Seafood 69

CHAPTER 6: Vegetables and Sides 85

CHAPTER 7: Desserts 105

MEASUREMENT CONVERSIONS **117**

INDEX **118**

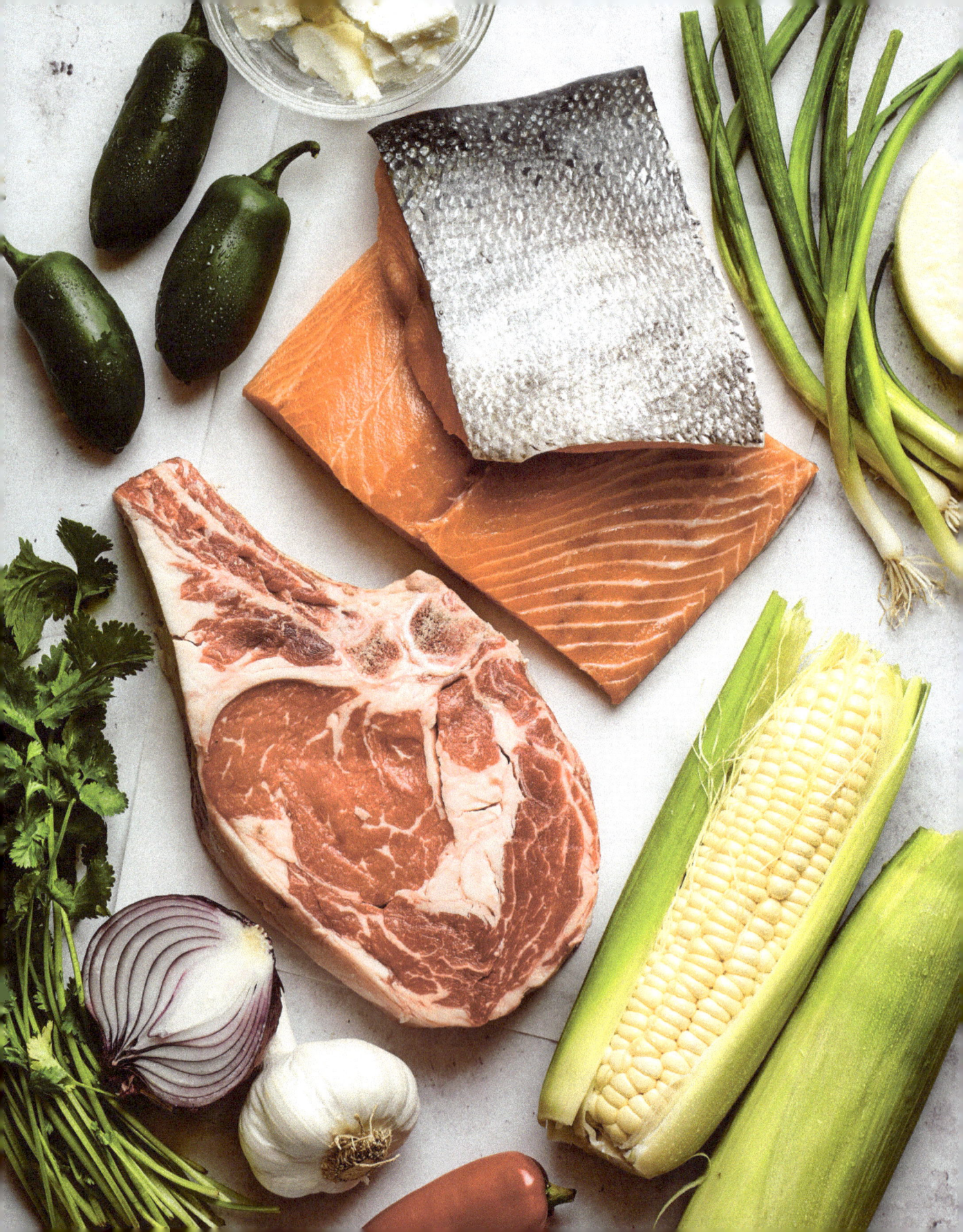

INTRODUCTION

I have been interested in cooking for as long as I can remember.
Growing up, I was always interested in what my mother was cooking and wanted to pitch in. During summer barbecues with my dad, I was fascinated by how fire could be used to cook such tasty meat. Later, I was exposed to many new cooking methods through cooking shows. I was mesmerized by Bobby Flay and his *Grillin' & Chillin'* series. That's when I was hooked. I figured if this guy from New York City could barbecue, then so could I. Over the next 10 years, with my wife, Vida, by my side, I attempted to perfect my craft, focusing on Kansas City and Texas barbecue styles. When we finally attended our first barbecue competition in 2009, I could not believe how openly the pitmasters shared their experiences and how happy they were to bring me behind the scenes and show me the magic that happened behind the curtain. Shortly after that experience, we started Revolution Barbecue, a barbecue spice rub company based in Thornton, Colorado. Our guiding idea was that no one type of barbecue was the right style, and our goal was to incorporate as many different styles as possible into our dishes—how revolutionary!

The last few years we have been living in Colorado, where we find ourselves enjoying the beautiful evenings and cooking outdoors nearly every day. Like most of you, we don't have time to fire up one of our smokers in the middle of the week and barbecue something for 12 hours. Like many home cooks, we generally have about an hour or less to prep and cook a weeknight meal. Our weekday struggles with the desire to barbecue and finding the time to do it were the foundation for this book.

This is more than just a collection of recipes; it is a journey through the techniques and tools needed to create great barbecue. These recipes are not just tried-and-true favorites but are also examples of skills you can apply to future recipes. If I accomplish anything with this book, I want to teach you the essentials of cooking over fire, so that every time you grill—whether you are making one of these recipes or one of your own—you possess the skills to succeed. You will be surprised how quickly your skills, along with your confidence, grow when you use these techniques.

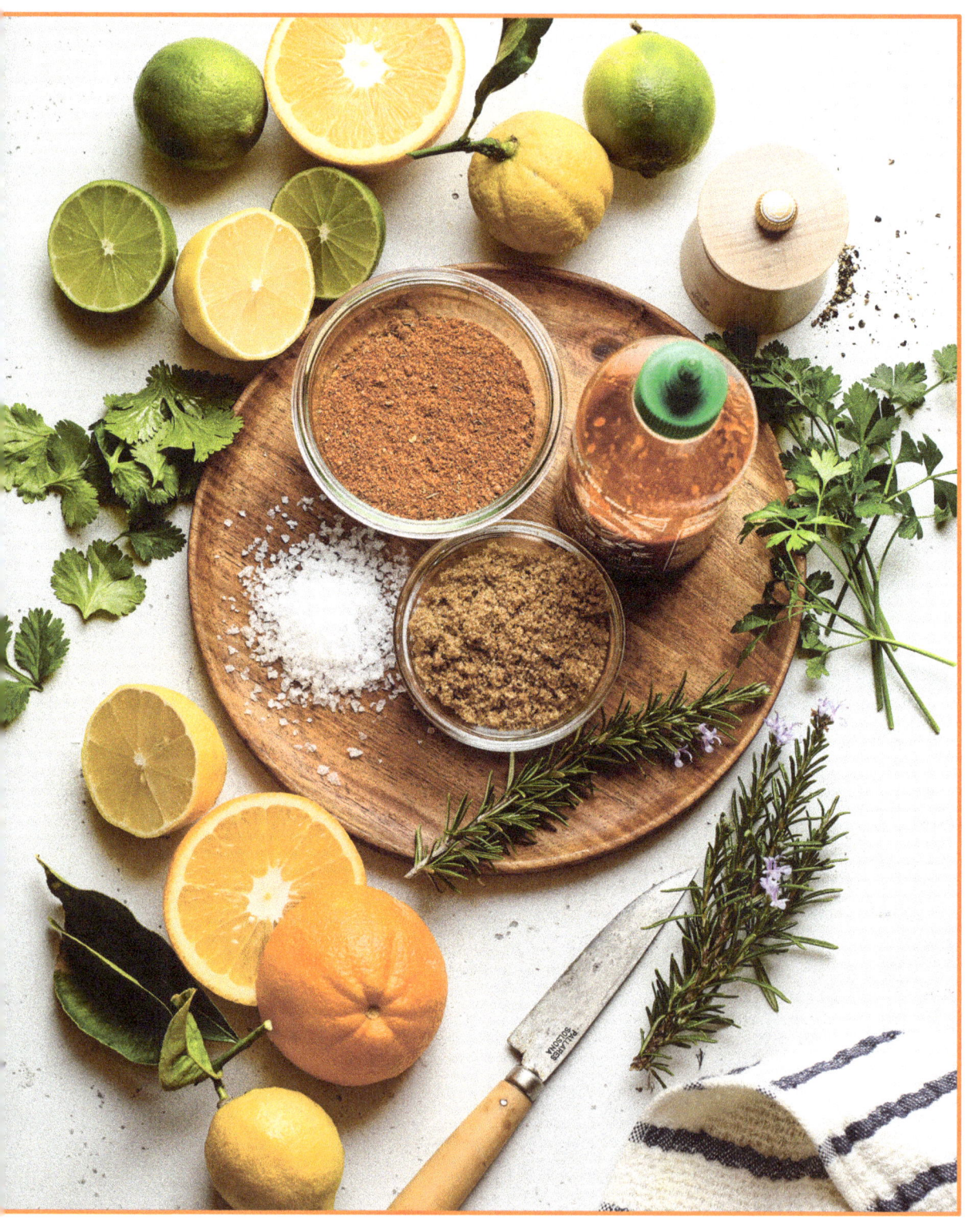

CHAPTER 1

EASY BBQ BASICS

STRATEGIES FOR MAKING BBQ EASY **2**

YOUR BBQ FLAVOR ARSENAL **3**

EQUIPPING YOUR EASY BBQ KITCHEN **7**

FIRE BASICS **8**

SMOKE IT EASY **13**

THE RECIPES **15**

STRATEGIES FOR MAKING BBQ EASY

Over the years, I have developed a variety of strategies for making barbecue easy. My approach is to keep my prep simple, focus on how using fewer ingredients and steps can actually result in more delicious meals, and employ some simple cheats to maximize my time.

The recipes in the following chapters utilize three methods of making barbecue on the grill: cooking with direct heat, indirect heat, and two-zone indirect heat. In this chapter, I'll explain those methods and how to use them. I'll also outline some basic tools of the trade that will let you master just about any dish.

In recent years, there has been an explosion of new barbecue gadgetry hitting the marketplace. I say avoid all this wizardry and stick with what has worked for decades. A simple multizone gas grill or a charcoal grill, along with a few basic tools, is all you need to turn out the most delicious barbecued meals.

Keep Prep Simple

A key to making barbecue easy is to be prepared before you start cooking. There is a French culinary term, *mise en place*, that is helpful to think about when preparing to make barbecue. The term simply means "everything in its place," and it refers to having all your ingredients assembled, measured, cut, peeled, etc., before you start cooking. By employing this technique, you will have all your tools and ingredients at the ready. The goal of this book is to show you that, for many dishes, you can do this prep in 15 minutes or fewer (usually while your grill is heating) and demonstrate how having your ingredients at the ready sets you up for success.

Less Is More

The recipes in this book are geared toward quick prep; they use a maximum of 10 ingredients and a total prep time of 15 minutes or fewer. Some recipes do require you to marinate the protein for a longer period for maximum flavor, but these marinades are easy to whip up; once they're ready, all you have to do is leave them to do their magic in the refrigerator. You'll also see how, with the right ingredients in your pantry, you can be ready to tackle these dishes without having to buy a huge arsenal of spices and specialty ingredients. On the next page, I list the ingredients that I always have in my pantry that allow me to whip up just about any barbecue dish, even when I'm in a hurry.

Cheats You'll Love

Throughout this book, I provide tips and cheats to simplify the cooking process and shorten the time you are tending the grill. You will learn to use the grill to do just what it was designed to do—add a smoky, grilled flavor to food—and use other tools, like your oven, to finish a meal and simplify the cooking process. The grill can also be a lot easier to use than you may think, and I will show you how to "set it and forget it" while you create fantastic meals. I will also show you how to master your ingredients, teaching you about the importance of bringing meats up to room temperature before grilling and pounding chicken breasts flat to ensure even cooking.

YOUR BBQ FLAVOR ARSENAL

In our home, we regularly cook from our pantry. We think about what protein to use for dinner, but often that is as far as our meal planning goes. We rely on the fact that we already have the basic ingredients we need to whip up just about any quick meal on a whim.

One of the most important parts of this pantry arsenal is our collection of spices. Having these spices at the ready is essential to a successful barbecue cook.

Salt

When cooking, I only use kosher salt or sea salt. Most table salt contains iodine, which can have a bitter taste when used in larger quantities. Most chefs prefer to use kosher salt, as it has a less intense salty flavor and is easy to pick up due to the size of the crystals. All references to salt in this book are to Diamond Crystal kosher salt unless otherwise specified. Note that Diamond Crystal salt crystals are nearly twice the size of other kosher salt crystals and that other brands, such as Morton, provide a very different level of saltiness. If you're not using Diamond Crystal kosher salt, start with half the amount of salt listed in the recipe to avoid oversalting your dishes. You can always add more later.

Black Pepper

Freshly ground black pepper is an essential ingredient in nearly every recipe I make. I suggest grinding black pepper just before you use it, as pepper oxidizes quickly and loses its potency and flavor over time.

Granulated Garlic

I prefer granulated garlic to powdered garlic as I find the powdered version is too intense; it also usually contains anticaking additives to keep it from clumping. (If you use powdered garlic in a spice rub, it will typically fall to the bottom of the mixture and will not distribute evenly on your meat.)

Granulated Onion

I also prefer granulated dried onion to powdered. The granulated version is less intense and mixes better with other spices.

Turbinado (Raw) Sugar

Adding sugar to barbecue rubs helps them form a crust on your meat. I prefer to use raw, unbleached sugar such as turbinado (also marketed as Sugar In The Raw). White granulated sugar is ground too finely for the intense heat of a typical barbecue grill and can burn easily, which adds a bitter flavor to food.

Brown Sugar

This essential ingredient is typically found in just about every barbecue rub recipe. I cook with both light and dark brown sugars, but if you are only going to have one on the shelf, I recommend light, as it is more universal. That said, the darker version has more of a molasses flavor and can add a bit of smokiness to your dish.

Vinegar

The acid in vinegar adds a zing of flavor to your barbecue and cuts the richness or sweetness of a dish. It also complements salt, creating a more balanced flavor. If you only have space for one type, my go-to is white vinegar as it has a more neutral flavor and doesn't change the flavor of a recipe. As white vinegar has a high acid level, add small amounts at a time until you reach your desired flavor. I also like to have apple cider vinegar around, as it is milder and sweeter and is good for barbecue sauces and mops or spritzes.

Canola Oil

I always have canola oil at the ready for grilling veggies, frying, or making dressings. It is a neutral oil with a high smoke point (meaning it can take higher temperatures than other oils without burning). You can also use vegetable, avocado, or safflower oil.

Lime Juice

Limes are great for adding flavor (and good for digestion), and their citric acid can help tenderize meats. If possible, always have fresh limes on hand to add to marinades, salsas, and sauces and to squeeze onto your grilled steaks and chicken. If using bottled lime juice, buy an all-natural lime juice without added sugar.

Cumin

This spice, with a warm, earthy taste with some notes of citrus, is quite popular in Southwestern- and Middle Eastern–inspired dishes. It works great on savory meats, like beef and lamb, and accentuates the sweetness of vegetables, like carrots and beets.

Kansas City–Style BBQ Sauce

A good Kansas City–style barbecue sauce is always good to have on hand. This sweet, tangy, ketchup-based sauce includes apple cider vinegar, brown sugar, cayenne, and molasses and is one of the most iconic barbecue flavors. This type of sauce dominates the grocery store shelves and, unless otherwise labeled, most barbecue sauces are modeled after this style of sauce. A balanced sauce will be a bit smoky and slightly sweet and have a touch of spice.

BBQ Rub

Being in the barbecue rub business, I never have a shortage of store-brand rubs in my pantry. A Kansas City–style rub, based on black pepper, cayenne pepper, paprika, salt, and sugar, is a good all-purpose mix for just about any protein, including fish. I also like to have a salt-based rub handy, which can have a pronounced salt and black pepper flavor profile and is usually mixed with garlic and other peppers. This type of rub is great on most heartier proteins, like beef or pork, and is also good for grilling vegetables. If you want to make your own rub, you can whip up this easy Homemade Barbecue Rub by mixing the following pantry ingredients:

2 tablespoons paprika

2 tablespoons kosher salt

2 tablespoons turbinado sugar

2 tablespoons brown sugar

1 tablespoon ground cumin

1 tablespoon granulated garlic

1 tablespoon granulated onion

1 teaspoon cayenne pepper

ADDING SMOKE WITHOUT FIRE

When we fire up our barbecue, we don't always have time to cook meat for hours and let it develop that deep smoky flavor we all love. Adding wood chips or pellets to your grill is a way to add smoke flavor to meat quickly. If you do not have wood chips or are looking to step up the smoke flavor even further, there are many spices that can also add some smoky flavor.

Chipotle: Chipotle chiles are smoke-dried jalapeños. These peppers come in several forms, including whole, powdered, and canned. Dried chipotle powder, which is available in most grocery store spice aisles, can be added to your barbecue rub to provide a spicy kick as well as a smoky flavor. Canned chipotles, which are softer, come mixed in adobo sauce, which can also be mixed with mayonnaise or ketchup to kick up flavor.

Smoked paprika: Paprika is a spice made from dried, ground peppers that originated in Central Mexico. Paprika is usually made from mild peppers and adds the same amount of spiciness to your food as black pepper. When choosing paprikas, you can opt for a sweet version, which is found in most barbecue rubs, or a smoked version that will add a touch of smokiness (as well as a beautiful red hue) to food.

Smoked salt: Salt smoked with mesquite or hickory can add a touch of smoky flavor to dishes. If using smoked salt, practice a "less is more" philosophy and add it to your food in small quantities until you reach your desired flavor. This way, you won't oversalt your food trying to get to the level of smokiness you want.

Liquid smoke: This flavor enhancer can be found in the spice aisle in most grocery stores, usually in either hickory or mesquite flavor. Believe it or not, liquid smoke is made from actual smoke and not chemicals. A wood fire is built and then the smoke is captured in condensers and combined with water. This spice is concentrated, and a little goes a long way: Use only a drop at a time in your marinade or sauce.

EQUIPPING YOUR EASY BBQ KITCHEN

There are an overwhelming number of grills and smokers on the market, and I will not attempt to go through all of them. I assume that if you have this book, you've already selected your favorite gas or charcoal grill and are ready to get grilling. The recipes in this book are geared toward using either a gas grill or a charcoal grill; you don't need a smoker or any other fancy equipment. In addition to a solid grill, there are some other tools that I feel are essential to a successful cook. Here are the tools I use every day to make barbecuing easier.

Wire Brush

A stiff, long-handled wire brush is an essential tool for cleaning a grill. Look for one that is sturdy enough to hold up to pressure when you apply some "elbow grease."

Chimney Lighter

A chimney lighter is a metal cylinder with a charcoal grate mounted toward the bottom that is designed to light a bunch of charcoal quickly and evenly, in about 15 minutes. Load the desired amount of charcoal into the chimney and light it using paper or starter cubes. Typical chimneys can load upward of 100 charcoal briquettes, which is enough to produce high heat in a standard grill for direct heat cooking.

Grill Pan

A grill pan is a sheet pan with small holes in it. It is quite useful for grilling vegetables or other smaller items, and using one can be a lot faster than skewering meats and vegetables. Look for a heavy-duty version that can take prolonged use over high heat. Avoid pans with Teflon or other nonstick coatings as the coatings will peel off over time, especially if used directly on the coals.

Disposable Aluminum Foil Pans

These 9-by-13-inch pans are some of the most indispensable barbecue multitaskers you can own: They can be used for marinating, cooking, and serving. Place wood chips in one, cover it with aluminum foil with holes poked in it, place it directly on your coals or gas burner, and it will turn your grill into a smoker. In my opinion, you can never have enough of these pans. Look for bulk packs in warehouse food stores for the best price.

Heavy-Duty Aluminum Foil

Aluminum foil is essential to backyard cooking, allowing you to cover meats while cooking, line grill grates, and make cooking packets. Be sure to use heavy-duty foil.

Spatula

I recommend that you have two spatulas: a smaller slotted turning spatula to move delicate items like fish, and a longer, heavy-duty version for heavier items.

Spring-Loaded Tongs

A good, sturdy pair of stainless-steel, long-handled tongs is essential for moving hot food around the grill. Look for tongs that have a locking mechanism for easy storage in your utensil drawer. If you have a charcoal grill, I recommend having a second pair to open the grill grate and move hot coals around to avoid contaminating your food with ash.

Meat Thermometer

Every cut of meat is different, and no amount of touching or poking will tell you if it is thoroughly and safely cooked. An instant-read thermometer takes instant temperature readings, within 2 to 3 seconds, and is meant to be removed after testing. Another option is a wireless thermometer that allows you to connect a temperature probe to a digital reader or your phone via Bluetooth or Wi-Fi.

Grill Gloves

Look for a glove that has a combination of cloth material and silicone grips and that can resist temperatures of at least 900°F. Unlike leather grilling gloves, the silicone coating allows you to grip cooking utensils easily.

FIRE BASICS

Knowing how to light your grill properly and maintain your desired temperature is fairly easy once you have some practice. These fundamentals will set you up for successful grilling, whether you are using a charcoal or a gas grill.

Lighting the Fire

Preheating the grill is critical to successful barbecue cooking. To preheat a gas grill, turn on all the burners to high heat (see below) and close the lid for 10 minutes. To preheat a charcoal grill, light the coals and wait until they are covered in white-gray ash, then pour them into your grill and cover it for at least 10 minutes. After preheating your grill, use a grill brush or long-handled tongs and a crumpled-up ball of aluminum foil to scrub the grill grates and remove any debris.

LIGHTING A GAS GRILL

1. Make sure all burners are in the off position before you start.
2. Open the propane tank fully to the "open" position, then lift the grill's lid.
3. Locate the ignition button on your grill, which is usually indicated by a lightning bolt or a flame. If the ignition button is not integrated into your temperature knob, turn the first burner knob to high and click the ignition button until the grill lights.
4. Continue this process for each burner until the grill is lit.
5. Close the lid and let the grill preheat and come to temperature.

Note: If a burner fails to light within the first 5 seconds, turn off the knob and let any gas escape before attempting to relight it.

If your gas grill requires you to start it with a lighter, remember to bring the gas to the flame and not the flame to the gas: To do this properly (and safely), place your stick lighter next to the burner and light it, then turn on the gas until the burner lights.

LIGHTING A CHARCOAL GRILL

1. Place two pieces of crumpled-up newspaper or two starter cubes (a natural, non-toxic tool for starting a charcoal fire made from a blend of wood and paraffin wax) under the charcoal chimney and place them on the charcoal grate (this is the grate toward the bottom of the grill, not the one on top where you place food).
2. Fill the chimney with charcoal: For high heat, fill the chimney completely; for medium-high, fill it three-fourths full; and for medium to low, fill it half full.
3. Light the paper or starter cubes using a long stick lighter or a long match. (I recommend that you never use lighter fluid or any other accelerant, including charcoal infused with lighting agents, as the fuel can put off an acrid smell that can

transfer to your food.) The coals will smoke heavily at first and then will begin to glow a deep orange-red color. Once this happens, pour the coals into the charcoal grate and let them continue to preheat until they begin to ash over.

4. Distribute the coals according to your cooking method (see instructions for Direct Fire, Indirect Fire, and Two-Zone cooking, opposite).

Gas Gauge Hack

Using a propane grill and worried you do not have sufficient gas in your tank? Pour 1 quart of hot tap water down the side of your propane tank, then run your hand down the side of the tank. The part of the tank at the top with no gas will be warm to the touch and the portion of the tank with the gas will be cold. Most tanks provide between 6 and 8 hours of grilling time.

CHARCOAL VERSUS BRIQUETTES AND BEYOND

The most popular fuel for a charcoal grill is charcoal briquettes. Most major name brands compress charcoal with a binding agent to make the briquette shape. In recent years, hardwood (or "lump charcoal") has increased in popularity. Lump charcoal is wood burned in a low-oxygen environment, producing larger chunks. Some believe that lump charcoal is "cleaner" as it has no binding agents, but both briquettes and lump charcoal start with scrap wood. Many tests show that briquettes burn just as hot, if not hotter, than lump charcoal and that they lasted upward of three times longer. In my opinion, you get a more consistent cook from uniform-size briquettes.

Cooks also have the option to use alternative types of charcoal from around the world. For authentic Japanese-style yakitori, for instance, you can use binchotan charcoal, which is made using ubame oak trees. For another regional favorite, try quebracho charcoal from South America, a dense hardwood that creates long-burning charcoal. One other charcoal worth mentioning is coconut shell charcoal. This charcoal puts off very little smoke and burns hotter and longer than traditional briquettes.

Direct Fire

Direct fire, or direct heat, cooking refers to the high heat grilling you typically use to sear a steak or grill a medium-rare burger. This cooking method is associated with those beautiful grill marks you expect from grilling and it leaves food moist and tender. This cooking method is ideal for foods seasoned with dry spices or rubs. When using the direct heat method, the food is cooked directly over the heat source, whether gas or charcoal. For either style of grill, the heat source only needs to be lit where the food is cooked. So, for a gas grill, only the burners directly under the food are lit. For a charcoal grill, push the charcoal to one side of the grill to concentrate the heat under the food.

Indirect Fire

Indirect fire, or indirect heat, cooking is typically used for low and slow cooking, for denser meats—such as roasts, turkey, or whole chickens—that need longer cooking times. If using a gas grill, turn on the burners on one side of the grill and cook the food over the unlit burners. When using a charcoal grill, push the coals to one side of the grill and place the food on the opposite side. When placing the lid on a charcoal grill, place the vents over the lit charcoal side, not the side where the food is, so the airflow passes over the coals rather than the food, keeping the temperature lower on the food side.

Two-Zone Indirect Fire

Two-zone indirect fire, or two-zone indirect heat, cooking is a combination of direct and indirect cooking methods. For this method, the gas burners or charcoal are lit only on one side of the grill, similar to the indirect fire method, but you cook on both sides of the grill. This cooking method is best for searing or reverse searing large chops or steaks: For the sear method, the meat is seared over direct heat on each side for 2 to 4 minutes and then moved to indirect heat to finish cooking. For the reverse sear method, the meat is cooked on the indirect heat side of the grill until it reaches a desired temperature of around 10°F to 15°F degrees less than your target temperature, then moved to direct heat to be seared until the desired temperate is reached. Much research has been done on whether it's better to sear or reverse sear meat, and experts agree that it's best to reverse sear large pieces of meat, as this brings up the internal temperature of the meat slowly, providing a more even cook and juicier results.

Maintaining Temperature

Whether using direct, indirect, or two-zone indirect methods, cooking at low, medium, medium-high, or high heat can mean a varying range of temperatures within each. Understanding these ranges will help you know if your temperature is correct.

TEMPERATURE RANGES FOR ALL BBQ COOKING STYLES	
Low Heat	225°F to 325°F
Medium Heat	325°F to 400°F
Medium-High Heat	400°F to 450°F
High Heat	450°F to 600°F

Regardless of the cooking style used, one of the biggest challenges when grilling is controlling the grill's temperature. Cooking at a consistent temperate ensures that food is cooked thoroughly and to your desired doneness.

★ With a gas grill with built-in gauges, this process is fairly straightforward. That said, not all grills are made the same. Become familiar with your gas grill and where the hot and cold zones are. On less-expensive gas grills, there can easily be 10°F to 20°F temperature differences between cooking zones.

★ On a charcoal grill, the first step is to make sure that you put food on the grill the moment the coals begin to ash over (roughly 20 minutes after they're lit). Depending on the cooking method you're using, you may need to rake the coals into a pile (which increases the temperature under the meat) or spread them out (which decreases the temperature).

★ When using charcoal, you can also use the vents on your grill to help control the temperature. Oxygen makes coals burn hotter, so leaving the vents open completely will increase the heat, whereas closing the vents will cool the coals.

★ If your grill has adjustable grates, you can increase the cooking temperature by lowering the grates to be closer to the heat or decrease the temperature by raising the grates.

Keep It Clean

Make sure your grill is thoroughly cleaned before use. A simple hack to clean a grill is to cover the entire surface of the grill grates with heavy-duty aluminum foil, set the grill to high heat, and close the lid. In about 5 minutes, the grill grates will be quite hot and ready to be cleaned. Carefully remove the foil and scrub the grill grates with a grill brush. If you do not have a grill brush, ball up the foil and use it as a brush to make your grates bright and shiny.

SMOKE IT EASY

Many cooks want to incorporate the flavor of smoke into their barbecue dishes. This is typically done by cooking foods low and slow for long periods in a smoker. But have no fear, a smoky flavor can also be achieved on your gas or charcoal grill. The introduction of smoke to your dish should be subtle and complement what you are cooking without overtaking it completely. Be sure to pair the proper wood with the dish you are cooking. You don't want a strong smoke flavor overpowering a delicate piece of salmon, for example. Here are the tools and steps you need to add a touch of smoke to your dishes (and impress your friends and family).

If you use wood chips or pellets, keep in mind that there is such a thing as too much smoke. When adding wood chips or pellets to your grill, use only a handful. If you need to add additional wood later, continue adding only a handful at a time. A clean smoke is described as a "thin blue line" rather than a thick cloud of black or white smoke. Wait for the smoke to dissipate before putting your food on the grill to avoid it taking on a harsh bitter flavor.

Fuel Options

If you're interested in smoking your foods, I suggest having three different flavors (in wood chips or 100-percent wood pellets) at the ready: For lighter dishes such as vegetables and fish, use apple wood, which has a lightly fruity smoke that will enhance these mild foods. For chicken, pork, and thinner beef cuts, I use hickory wood, which puts off a stronger smoke flavor but is not overpowering. Lastly, for thicker cuts of beef such as cowboy steaks, I suggest mesquite wood. This is the flavor most associated with Texas-style barbecue and is also the most smoke-forward option.

CHIPS AND CHUNKS

There are typically two types of wood used for smoking: Larger wood chunks are usually used in a smoker while cooking low and slow, whereas smaller wood chips are perfect in a barbecue grill. (See How to Smoke on a Charcoal Grill, below.)

FOOD-GRADE WOOD PELLETS

With the huge rise in popularity of pellet smokers, there is an abundance of wood pellets on the market these days. Look for a wood pellet made from 100-percent hardwood in the flavor you desire. Some manufacturers use natural hardwood, such as alder, and then use oil to flavor them, which should be avoided.

How to Smoke on a Charcoal Grill

It is quite easy to have your charcoal grill put off a whisper of smoke to enhance foods. One way to achieve this is to toss some wood chips directly onto the charcoal while preheating the grill, which gives them time to burn down a bit and start to put off smoke. Make sure that the wood chips are putting off a bluish, or "clean," smoke and not a cloud of white or black smoke. A bluish smoke means that the wood is at the proper temperature for flavoring your meat. If your wood chips are putting off black smoke, they are not ready and will put off soot and an acrid flavor.

KEEPING IT DRY OR WET

One of the greatest myths about barbecuing is the need to soak wood chips before smoking with them. Much research has been done on this subject, and experts have found that if you wet the wood, you end up with steam instead of the smoke you want. Here's what happens: Most fruitwoods, nut woods, and other hardwoods used for cooking have a very tight grain and contain only about 10 percent moisture, making it nearly impossible for water to penetrate the wood. Water boils at 212°F. When you place the wood on about 600°F coals, once the water reaches the boiling point, it will steam. For wood to put off smoke, it needs to reach its combustion point of roughly 575°F. So, if you soaked the wood, the evaporating water will put off steam instead of smoke and keep the wood from smoking properly. Simply put: Don't do it.

How to Smoke on a Gas Grill

You can also introduce smoke into your dishes on a gas grill. Many manufacturers now add a smoke drawer to their grills. I like having the smoke drawer on one end, so as not to interfere with indirect cooking, but most models have the drawer in the center of the grill. There are also some other tools available:

★ **Smoke Box:** A smoke box is a small metal container that can be placed directly on a burner. Place your favorite wood chips inside, put the box on top of the burner, and turn the flame to high until the chips put off bluish smoke, then turn the burner down. I prefer to put the smoke box on the far side of the grill, so it does not interfere with any indirect grilling.

★ **Smoke Tubes:** A smoke tube is very similar to a smoke box but is shaped like a tube and is typically used with wood pellets. Fill the smoke tube with pellets and place it directly on the burner. Light the burner and let the pellets burn for about 5 minutes. Turn off the burner and blow out any flame in the smoke tube. You are now ready to cook as planned and infuse your dish with smoke.

★ **Smoke Packets:** If you do not have any of the fancy accessories listed above, you can easily create an aluminum foil smoke packet. Place a good handful of wood chips into the middle of a sheet of foil. Fold all four sides of the foil over the wood chips to completely enclose them and tightly seal the foil. Using a knife, puncture the foil packet 10 times to let smoke escape. Place the packet directly on the burner and light it on high heat until the wood puts off a bluish smoke. Reduce the heat to low, and the packet will continue to put off smoke.

THE RECIPES

The recipes in this book are a compilation of dishes I cook regularly for my family. If you are like me and have a busy schedule, taking a long time to prep meals is typically unrealistic, so I have brought together recipes that use 10 ingredients or fewer and can be prepped in about 30 minutes. There is a blend of classic and contemporary recipes that are influenced by flavors from around the world. I have put my spin on several traditional dishes by adapting them for the grill and reducing the number of steps needed to make them. Throughout this book, look for EZ BBQ tips, which show you how to shorten cook times and introduce useful tools, and variation tips, which will help you put your own spin on these dishes.

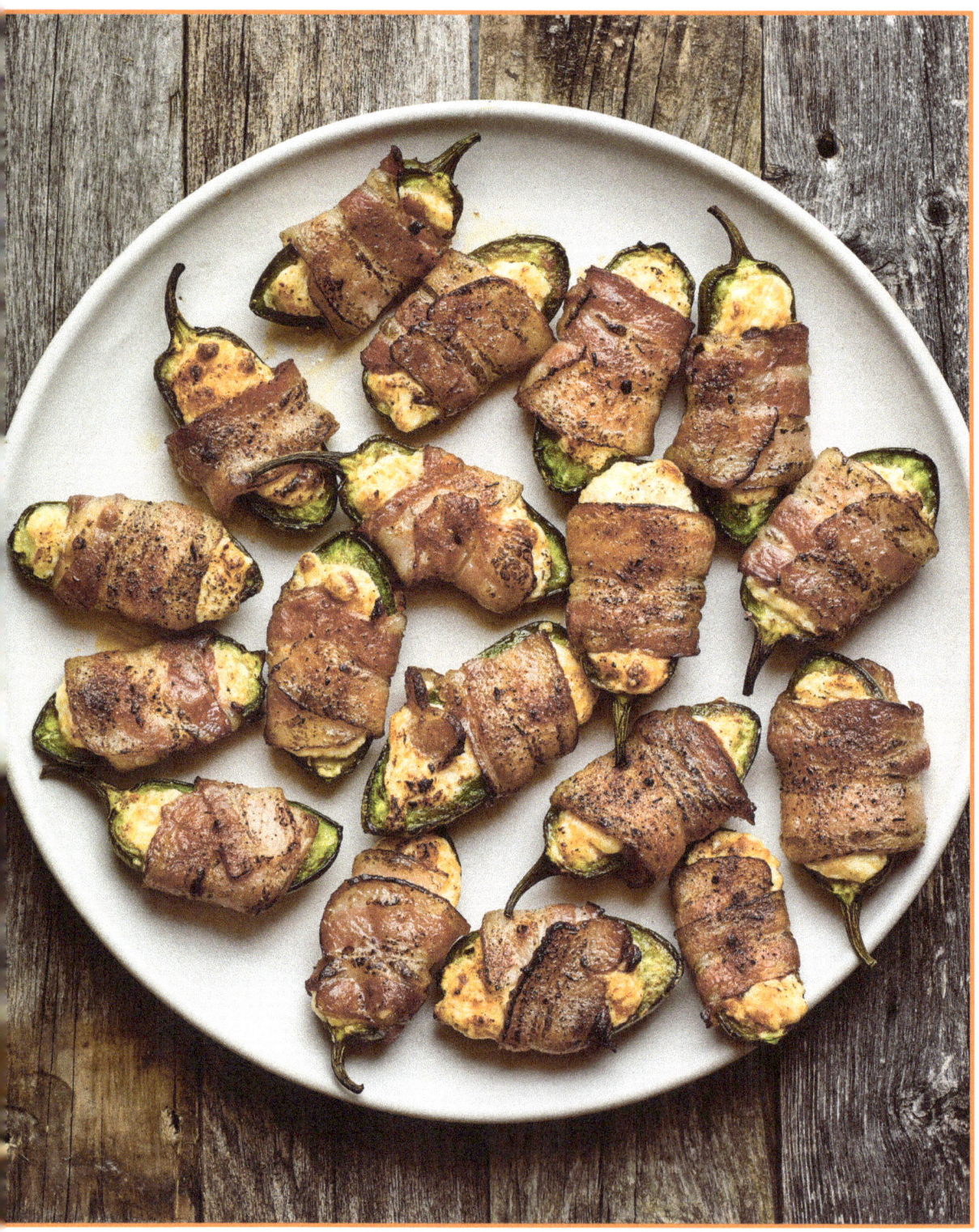

CHAPTER 2

APPETIZERS

★ BACON-WRAPPED JALAPEÑO POPPERS **19** ★

FIRE-ROASTED SALSA **20**

JALAPEÑO-CHEESE SKILLET DIP **21**

MOINK BALLS **22**

GRILLED WATERMELON WEDGES **23**

SMOKED DEVILED EGGS **24**

APPETIZERS CHEAT SHEET

Often overlooked when it comes to barbecuing, grilled appetizers can often be made on an unused portion of the grill while you're cooking the main dish.

BBQ COOKING STYLES

Direct heat:
400°F to 425°F, medium-high heat
600°F, high heat

Indirect heat:
250°F, low heat
350°F, medium heat

USEFUL TOOLS

Pizza stone: This slab distributes heat evenly and can be placed directly on your grill. In addition to making pizza, it is great for quesadillas, frozen French fries, and grilling bread. You can also crisp oiled chicken skin directly on the stone.

Cast-iron skillet: A cast-iron skillet is one of the best multitasking cooking tools you can have. When properly seasoned, cast iron requires little to no oil or butter to prevent foods from sticking. It heats evenly and holds its temperature, which is ideal for cooking over fire.

KEEP IN MIND

Keep it clean. As appetizers are the first dish of the meal, they may be the first foods on the grill; make sure your grill is cleaned before you begin cooking.

COMMON PROBLEMS

Undercooked bacon: Some of the tastiest grilled appetizers have an outer layer of bacon. To prevent undercooked bacon, use standard or thin-cut bacon. Thick-cut bacon is often still soggy, instead of crisp, when the other ingredients are cooked.

BACON-WRAPPED JALAPEÑO POPPERS

DIRECT HEAT COOKING
MAKES 16 POPPERS ★ **PREP TIME:** 15 MINUTES ★ **COOK TIME:** 20 MINUTES
TOOLS: Toothpicks

This is one of my absolute favorite BBQ appetizers! Here, jalapeños are stuffed with melty cheese and then wrapped in bacon. What else do you need? For this recipe, I use a shredded Mexican cheese blend, which usually contains cheddar, Monterey Jack, asadero, and queso quesadilla cheeses.

- 8 jalapeño peppers
- 8 ounces cream cheese, at room temperature
- ½ cup shredded Mexican cheese blend
- 8 bacon slices, halved widthwise
- 2 tablespoons Homemade Barbecue Rub (page 5) or store-bought
- 2 tablespoons canola oil

1. Preheat the grill to medium-high heat (425°F) for direct heat cooking by lighting the heat source (or piling coals) in the spot that will be directly under the food.

2. Cut off the stems of the jalapeños and halve them lengthwise. Using a teaspoon, scrape out the seeds and the white membrane. In a small bowl, combine the cream cheese and the cheese blend and mix well. Spoon equal portions of the cheese mixture into the jalapeño halves.

3. Wrap each jalapeño half with a half slice of bacon, securing it with a toothpick. (If you do not have toothpicks, make sure the ends of the bacon overlap on the bottom of the pepper, not against the cheese.) Sprinkle the rub over the wrapped poppers.

4. Put the oil on a folded paper towel and use a large pair of tongs to wipe down the grill grate with it.

5. Place the jalapeños on the grill, cheese-side down, and cook for about 6 minutes, or until the bacon gets crispy. Using long-handled tongs, carefully flip the poppers.

6. Reduce the heat to medium (350°F) and cook for 10 to 12 minutes, or until the bacon is crisp on all sides.

FIRE-ROASTED SALSA

DIRECT HEAT COOKING

MAKES 8 CUPS ★ **PREP TIME:** 15 MINUTES + 1 HOUR TO CHILL ★ **COOK TIME:** 15 MINUTES

We've been making this family favorite for more than 25 years. We even won a salsa competition with a superhot variation of this salsa. I use Roma tomatoes because of their low water content and meaty texture. You can use other tomatoes, but you may need to drain them before grilling. This salsa is best after it has chilled for at least an hour in the refrigerator.

- 2 tablespoons canola oil
- 2½ pounds Roma tomatoes
- 2 jalapeño peppers
- 2 medium sweet onions
- ¼ cup chopped fresh cilantro
- Juice of 1 lime
- 2 tablespoons white vinegar
- 1½ teaspoons kosher salt
- 1 teaspoon freshly ground black pepper

1. Preheat the grill to high heat (600°F) for direct heat cooking by lighting the heat source (or piling coals) in the spot that will be directly under the food. Put the oil on a folded paper towel and use a large pair of tongs to wipe down the grill grate with it.

2. Remove the stems from the tomatoes and jalapeños. Quarter the onions from top to bottom, leaving the bases intact so the wedges do not fall apart.

3. Place the tomatoes, jalapeños, and onions on the grill. Cook for about 7 minutes, until the tomatoes are charred and slightly split. Flip the vegetables using long-handled tongs. Grill for 7 minutes more, or until the tomatoes are charred and soft. Remove the vegetables from the grill.

4. Cut off the bases from the onions (careful, they are hot).

5. Working in batches, put equal amounts of the grilled vegetables into a food processor and pulse until chunky. Pour the contents into a large bowl. Repeat with the remaining grilled vegetables until they are all chopped.

6. Add the cilantro, lime juice, vinegar, salt, and pepper and stir until fully incorporated.

7. Refrigerate the salsa for at least 1 hour to allow the flavors to meld and mature.

JALAPEÑO-CHEESE SKILLET DIP

INDIRECT HEAT COOKING
SERVES 4 ★ **PREP TIME:** 10 MINUTES ★ **COOK TIME:** 30 MINUTES
TOOLS: Apple or hickory wood chips (optional), cast-iron skillet

An easy-to-make crowd-pleaser, this dip can be cooked in advance and reheated in a 350°F oven for about 15 minutes. Add some smoky flavor by putting some apple or hickory wood chips in your grill while it's preheating.

- 8 ounces cream cheese, at room temperature
- 1 (8-ounce) block pepper Jack cheese, shredded, divided
- 1 (8-ounce) block sharp cheddar cheese, shredded
- ⅓ cup mayonnaise
- 4 teaspoons taco seasoning, divided
- 3 jalapeño peppers, seeded and finely chopped
- Corn chips or tortilla chips, for serving

1. Preheat the grill to medium heat (350°F) for indirect heat cooking by lighting only the heat source (or piling coals) across from where you will place the food. Add a handful of apple or hickory wood chips to the grill (if using).

2. In a medium bowl, stir together the cream cheese, half of the pepper Jack cheese, the cheddar, mayonnaise, and 2 teaspoons of taco seasoning until fully incorporated. Spread the cheese mixture into a cast-iron skillet. Sprinkle the top of the mixture with the jalapeños, the remaining pepper Jack, and the remaining 2 teaspoons of taco seasoning.

3. Place the skillet on the grill opposite the heat and close the lid. Cook for 25 to 30 minutes, until the cheese is hot and bubbly.

4. Serve warm with chips for dipping.

VARIATION TIP: For a creamy version with an added bit of tang, add 1 cup of sour cream to the cheese mixture in step 2.

APPETIZERS

MOINK BALLS

DIRECT HEAT COOKING
MAKES 16 BALLS ★ **PREP TIME:** 15 MINUTES ★ **COOK TIME:** 30 MINUTES
TOOLS: Hickory or mesquite wood chips (optional), toothpicks

Back in the early 2000s, when we were on the competition BBQ circuit, this dish was a staple of the BBQ scene. Just about every team would hand it out to the public for the People's Choice Awards. For an added smoky flavor, add hickory or mesquite wood to your grill when preheating it.

- 1 pound ground beef (80% lean, 20% fat)
- ½ cup plain bread crumbs
- ¼ cup freshly grated Parmesan cheese
- 1 large egg
- 1 tablespoon Homemade Barbecue Rub (page 5) or store-bought
- 1 teaspoon minced garlic
- 8 bacon slices, halved widthwise
- 1 cup barbecue sauce, warmed

1. Preheat the grill to medium-high heat (400°F) for direct heat cooking by lighting the heat source (or piling coals) in the spot that will be directly under the food. Add a handful of hickory or mesquite wood chips to the grill (if using).

2. In a medium bowl, mix the ground beef, bread crumbs, Parmesan, egg, barbecue rub, and garlic until well mixed. (Don't overwork the meat or the balls will be tough.) Roll the meat into roughly 1½-ounce meatballs, about the size of a golf ball. Wrap each meatball with a half slice of bacon and secure it with a toothpick.

3. Place the meatballs on the grill grate and cook them for 15 minutes. The meatballs will show signs of browning and the bacon will begin to tighten. Use a pair of long-handled tongs to gently flip the meatballs. Cook for 15 minutes, or until the bacon has rendered its fat and is slightly crispy.

4. Remove the meatballs from the grill and place them in a medium bowl. Add the barbecue sauce and toss well to coat. Remove the meatballs from the bowl and serve warm.

EZ BBQ TIP: If you are in a hurry, use premade meatballs from your grocery store. The Italian-flavored varieties marry well with the bacon and barbecue sauce. Just thaw them thoroughly before cooking, so the bacon doesn't get soggy.

GRILLED WATERMELON WEDGES

DIRECT HEAT COOKING
SERVES 4 ★ **PREP TIME:** 10 MINUTES ★ **COOK TIME:** 10 MINUTES

Looking for an appetizer that is super easy and will blow everyone's socks off? This grilled watermelon with balsamic vinegar and feta cheese is just the thing. I know you are telling yourself there is no way this will work, but once you try it, you will never want to eat plain watermelon again. For the balsamic vinegar, splurge a bit and get the good stuff, which will be stamped with the mark DOP, which stands for Denominazione di Origine Protetta (or "Protected Designation of Origin").

2 tablespoons canola oil
1 (3-pound) watermelon (seedless preferred)
¼ cup balsamic vinegar
1 cup feta cheese crumbles
12 fresh mint leaves, chopped
Grated zest of 1 lemon

1. Preheat the grill to medium-high heat (425°F) for direct heat cooking by lighting the heat source (or piling coals) in the spot that will be directly under the food. Put the oil on a folded paper towel and use a large pair of tongs to wipe down the grill grate with it.

2. Slice the watermelon into 2-inch-thick rounds. Slice each round into 4 wedges. Place the watermelon slices on the grill and cook them for about 4 minutes, until grill marks develop. Flip the slices and repeat the process on the other side.

3. Transfer the watermelon slices to a platter and drizzle them lightly with the vinegar. Sprinkle on the feta crumbles and top with the mint and lemon zest.

EZ BBQ TIP: If you find that your watermelon is not quite ripe or lacking flavor, sprinkle a few pinches of kosher salt onto its flesh. The salt brings out the fruit's natural sweetness.

SMOKED DEVILED EGGS

STOVETOP + INDIRECT HEAT COOKING
MAKES 18 DEVILED EGGS ★ **PREP TIME:** 15 MINUTES ★ **COOK TIME:** 45 MINUTES
TOOLS: Hickory or mesquite wood chips, piping bag with large tip

This recipe takes a total of 1 hour to complete, but the results are worth the time invested. These eggs have tang from the yellow mustard, saltiness from the bacon, sweetness from the BBQ rub, and spice from the jalapeños, along with an infusion of smoke. Once you try these eggs, you will never want plain deviled eggs again.

- 9 large eggs
- 2 bacon slices, finely chopped
- 1 jalapeño pepper
- ⅓ cup mayonnaise
- 2 teaspoons Homemade Barbecue Rub (page 5), Kansas City–style barbecue rub, or store-bought, plus more for topping
- 1½ teaspoons white vinegar
- 1½ teaspoons yellow mustard
- 3 scallions, white and green parts, coarsely chopped

1. Fill a medium pot with water, place it over medium-high heat on the stovetop, and bring the water to a boil. Use a serving spoon to gently place the eggs in the water and cook for 9 minutes. Drain the water and rinse the eggs in cold water until cool enough to handle. Peel the eggs and halve them lengthwise.

2. Preheat the grill to low heat (250°F) for indirect grilling by lighting the heat source (or piling coals) on one side of the grill. Add a handful of hickory or mesquite wood chips to the grill.

3. Scoop out the yolks from the eggs and place them in a small bowl. Place the egg whites on the indirect side of the grill (away from the heat), close the lid, and smoke for 30 minutes. Meanwhile, in a sauté pan or skillet over medium-high heat on the stovetop, cook the bacon for 8 to 9 minutes, until crispy. Remove the bacon from the pan.

4. Remove the stem from the jalapeño, halve it lengthwise, and scoop out the seeds and membrane. Finely chop the pepper. Add the jalapeño to the bowl with the egg yolks along with the mayonnaise, barbecue rub, vinegar, and mustard. Using a fork, mash the mixture until smooth.

5. Using a teaspoon or a piping bag with a large tip, fill each egg white half with equal amounts (2 to 3 teaspoons) of the yolk mixture.

6. Top each egg half with a sprinkle of barbecue rub and equal amounts of the bacon and scallions.

VARIATION TIP: For a healthier version of this dish, substitute a ripe avocado mashed with 1 tablespoon of light sour cream for the mayonnaise. Mix these substitutes with the remaining ingredients in step 4.

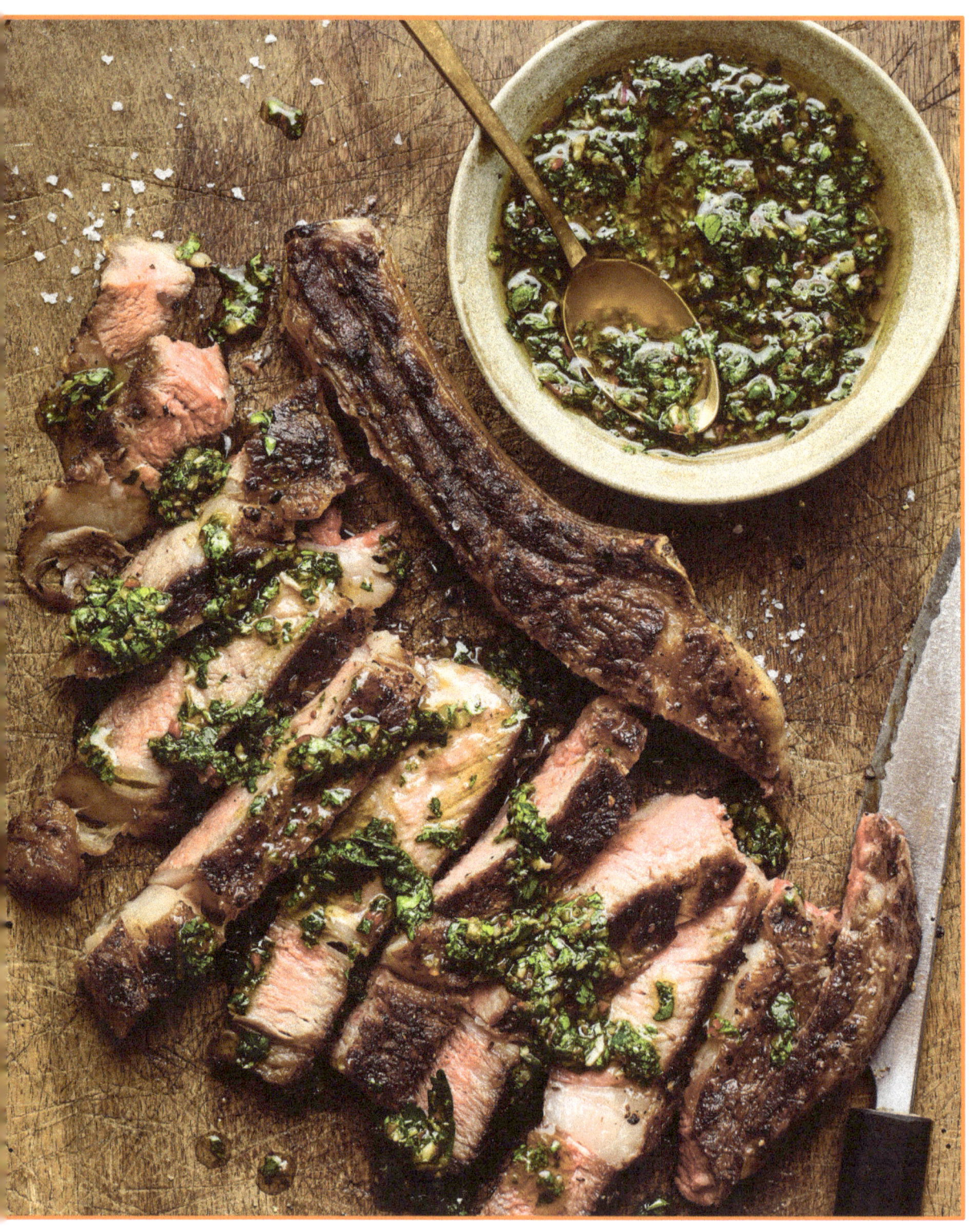

CHAPTER 3

BEEF AND PORK

BACON SMASH BURGERS **30**

CHEESY MEAT LOAF "PARMESAN" **32**

GRILLED SANTA MARIA–STYLE TRI-TIP **34**

BEEF SHORT RIBS **35**

GRILLED BEEF FAJITA SALAD WITH CILANTRO-LIME DRESSING **36**

★ REVERSE SEARED COWBOY STEAK WITH CHIMICHURRI SAUCE **38** ★

KOREAN-STYLE SHORT RIBS **41**

GRILLED AL PASTOR SKEWERS **42**

MAPLE-BOURBON PORK CHOPS WITH SMOKED APPLESAUCE **44**

CHAR SIU PORK TENDERLOIN **46**

MEAT CHEAT SHEET

One of America's favorite pastimes is grilling up a big chunk of meat; with the right setup, you can make anything from quick steaks or burgers to tender smoked ribs.

BBQ COOKING STYLES

Direct heat:
325°F to 350°F, medium heat
450°F, medium-high heat
500°F to 600°F, high heat

Indirect heat:
325°F, medium heat

Two-zone indirect heat:
350°F, medium heat
450°F, medium-high heat
500°F, high heat

INTERNAL TEMPS

FOOD TYPE	INTERNAL TEMPS			
Beef Steaks, Tri-Tips, Smaller Roasts	125°F: rare	135°F: med-rare	145°F: medium,	160°F: well-done
Pork Chops and Roasts	145°F: USDA-recommended safe temperature	135°F to 145°F: med-rare	145°F to 155°F: medium	155°F or higher: well-done
Briskets, Pork Shoulders, Rump Roasts	195°F to 205°F: to break down collagen for tender slices or pulling the meat			

USEFUL TOOLS

Instant-read thermometer: Using a thermometer is the single best thing you can do to achieve a perfect cook. No amount of poking at or squeezing will ever really tell you when the meat is cooked.

KEEP IN MIND

Don't forget to rest. Resting meat is an important step in the cooking process. It is tempting to take meat right from the grill and devour it, but resting the meat for a few minutes after cooking allows the juices to redistribute, creating a juicier and more tender dish.

Oil is your friend. For many recipes, it is critical to oil either the grill grates or the meat to prevent the meat from sticking to the grill. A small amount of oil is all it takes and it will not alter the dish's flavor. I typically use canola oil for most recipes, as it has a neutral flavor and a high smoke point, which keeps it from burning.

Meat temperature matters. For thicker cuts of meat, let them come to room temperature before grilling. The center of the meat will come up to temperature faster if it starts cooking when at room temperature, leading to less moisture loss while cooking for a more even cook and juicier meat.

COMMON PROBLEMS

Under seasoning: Many cuts of meat are fairly large and can take a heavy application of spice. Think about the way you are going to cut the meat and how much surface area will have the seasoning on it. Most of the spices applied to the meat will only be on the surface and will not penetrate into the interior of the cut.

ALSO TRY

Unless you're applying a sauce to your meat, **add a few pats of butter** right at the end of cooking; it will combine with the meat's juices and enhance the flavor. The butter can be added to the meat during the last minute of cooking or placed on your resting plate, with the meat on top of it.

BACON SMASH BURGERS

DIRECT HEAT COOKING
MAKES 4 BURGERS ★ **PREP TIME:** 15 MINUTES ★ **COOK TIME:** 7 MINUTES
TOOLS: Cast-iron skillet, griddle, or flat top grill accessory

In my opinion, there is nothing better than a smash burger—except a smash burger with a crust that is amped up with bacon. A smash burger is just what it sounds like: a burger that is smashed on a flattop or griddle. This process provides maximum crust and maximum flavor. Feel free to choose any good melting cheese for your burger, but I recommend American because it melts quickly and has a creamy texture.

FOR THE SAUCE
½ cup mayonnaise
¼ cup ketchup
1 tablespoon sweet or kosher pickle relish
2 teaspoons white vinegar
1 teaspoon freshly ground black pepper
1 teaspoon granulated garlic

FOR THE BURGERS
1 pound ground beef chuck (80% lean, 20% fat)
6 bacon slices, finely chopped
1 teaspoon kosher salt
1 teaspoon freshly ground black pepper
4 brioche buns
4 slices cheese of choice
Sliced red onion, for serving (optional)
Pickles, for serving (optional)

1. Preheat the grill to high heat (600°) for direct heat cooking by lighting the heat source (or piling coals) in the spot that will be directly under the food.

2. Place a cast-iron skillet on the grill and let it get hot for about 15 minutes.

3. Meanwhile, in a small bowl, stir together the mayonnaise, ketchup, relish, vinegar, pepper, and garlic until the sauce is well mixed

4. Divide the ground beef into four equal portions and form each into a ball. Spread the bacon on a plate. Roll the ball-shaped patties in the bacon until they are completely covered, then sprinkle them with the salt and pepper.

5. Quickly toast the buns on the grill, cut-side down, for 1 to 2 minutes, then transfer them to a plate.

6. Place the bacon-burger patties in the hot skillet and let them sit for 1 minute. Then, use a heavy metal spatula to smash down the burgers into thin patties. Cook for about 2 minutes, until a crust forms on the bottom. Flip the patties and top them with the cheese. Cook for 2 minutes more, until a crust forms on the bottom and the cheese melts.

7. Remove the burgers from the grill and place one on each bun. Serve with the sauce, red onion (if using), and pickles (if using).

EZ BBQ TIP: When you are just about to finish smashing your burger, slide the spatula horizontally off the meat so it doesn't stick. If it still sticks, you can use a small piece of parchment paper or aluminum foil between the spatula and the meat.

CHEESY MEAT LOAF "PARMESAN"

STOVETOP + INDIRECT HEAT COOKING
SERVES 6 ★ PREP TIME: 15 MINUTES ★ **COOK TIME:** 45 MINUTES

This is no ordinary meat loaf. This cheesy dish is a play on an Italian classic, chicken Parmigiana, overhauled and reimagined as a beef and sausage meat loaf. It consists of ground beef and Italian sausage, along with bread crumbs, and it is topped with marinara sauce and mozzarella cheese. The meat is also flavored with Italian seasoning, which typically consists of basil, thyme, oregano, marjoram, and rosemary.

- 1 tablespoon canola oil
- 1 medium sweet onion, finely chopped
- 2 celery stalks, finely chopped
- 2 garlic cloves, minced
- 1½ pounds ground beef (80% lean, 20% fat)
- 8 ounces Italian sausage, removed from the casing, if needed
- 1 cup Italian bread crumbs
- 2 large eggs, beaten
- 2 tablespoons Italian seasoning
- 2 tablespoons Worcestershire sauce
- 1 teaspoon freshly ground black pepper
- 1 teaspoon kosher salt
- 1¼ cups shredded mozzarella cheese, divided
- 1 cup marinara sauce

1. Place a sauté pan or skillet over medium-high heat on the stovetop and pour in the oil. Add the onion, celery, and garlic and cook for about 5 minutes, stirring frequently, until translucent and soft. Remove the mixture from the heat and let cool.

2. Preheat the grill to medium heat (350°F) for indirect heat cooking by lighting only the heat source (or piling coals) across from where you will place the food.

3. While the grill preheats, in a large bowl, combine the cooked vegetable mixture, ground beef, sausage, bread crumbs, eggs, Italian seasoning, Worcestershire sauce, pepper, salt, and ½ cup of mozzarella.

4. Stack two 12-by-18 inch sheets of heavy-duty aluminum foil. Place the meat mixture in the middle of the foil and use your hands to form it into a loaf about 3 inches wide, 3 inches tall, and 12 inches long. Pour the marinara over the loaf and top it with the remaining ¾ cup of mozzarella. Fold up 1 inch of the foil along all sides to create a makeshift baking sheet (this will prevent grease from dripping onto your grill).

5. Place the foil sheets with the meat loaf on the indirect side of the grill, close the lid, and cook for 20 minutes. Rotate the foil 180 degrees, close the grill, and cook for 20 minutes more. The meat loaf is done when the cheese is browned and the internal temperature reaches 160°F.

6. Remove the meat loaf from the grill by carefully sliding the foil onto a baking sheet. Let rest for 10 minutes before slicing and serving.

VARIATION TIP: I use marinara sauce in this recipe, but feel free to experiment with any other flavor of pasta sauce. Some of my favorites are a triple-cheese pasta sauce, which adds to the cheesiness of the dish, and a roasted garlic pasta sauce, which complements the garlic in the meat loaf.

GRILLED SANTA MARIA-STYLE TRI-TIP

TWO-ZONE INDIRECT HEAT COOKING

SERVES 4 ★ **PREP TIME:** 10 MINUTES + 15 MINUTES TO REST ★ **COOK TIME:** 40 MINUTES

My family and I learned about tri-tip while living in Southern California. It is a triangular-shaped piece of beef that is sliced from the top sirloin and typically weighs 2 to 3 pounds. Given how tender and delicious this cut of beef is, I would lean toward 8 to 12 ounces per person as a serving size.

- 1½ tablespoons light brown sugar
- 1½ tablespoons smoked paprika
- 1 tablespoon ground cumin
- 1 tablespoon kosher salt
- 2 teaspoons freshly ground black pepper
- 2 teaspoons chili powder
- 1 teaspoon granulated garlic
- 1 teaspoon granulated onion
- ½ teaspoon cayenne pepper
- 2 to 3 pounds tri-tip
- 1 teaspoon canola oil

1. In a small bowl, stir together the brown sugar, paprika, cumin, salt, black pepper, chili powder, garlic, onion, and cayenne. Trim away any silver skin (the thin, fibrous membrane on the meat) and any chunks of fat on the tri-tip. Rub the tri-tip all over with the oil. Season the meat liberally with the spice rub (reserve any remaining rub). Let the meat rest while you prepare the grill.

2. Preheat the grill to medium-high heat (450°F) for two-zone indirect heat cooking by lighting the heat source (or piling coals) on one side of the grill.

3. Place the meat on the direct heat side of the grill, directly over the flame or the hot coals, with the lid open. Sear for 5 minutes, then flip the meat and sear the other side for 5 minutes.

4. Move the meat to the indirect heat side of the grill. Close the grill lid and cook the tri-tip for 20 to 30 minutes, or until the interior temperature reaches 5°F less than your desired doneness, so 120°F for a rare roast, 130°F for medium-rare, and 140°F for medium. Remove the tri-tip from the grill and let it rest, wrapped loosely with aluminum foil, for 15 minutes. (The carryover heat will increase the final temperature by 5°F while resting.) Do not discard the juices.

5. Slice the meat across the grain into ¼-inch-thick slices. Place the sliced meat back into the juices that were collected in the foil and serve.

BEEF SHORT RIBS

INDIRECT HEAT COOKING
SERVES 4 ★ **PREP TIME:** 5 MINUTES + 20 MINUTES TO REST ★ **COOK TIME:** 5 HOURS
TOOLS: Cherry or oak wood chips (optional)

There is nothing more sumptuous than perfectly prepared beef short ribs. They are simpler to cook than a brisket, consistent in their size, and have more fat (also known as flavor) than a rib eye. This recipe uses what is typically referred to as "English cut" short ribs, which are cut parallel to the bone and then cut in half, with the ribs being 2 to 3 inches in length. They should have a single bone going through the meat. A simple application of salt, pepper, and garlic is all you need to accentuate these ribs.

- 8 (3-ounce) English cut bone-in beef short ribs
- 3 tablespoons vinegar-based hot sauce
- 2 tablespoons kosher salt
- 2 tablespoons freshly ground black pepper
- 1 tablespoon granulated garlic

1. Preheat the grill to medium heat (325°F) for indirect heat cooking by lighting only the heat source (or piling coals) across from where you will place the food. Add a handful of cherry or oak wood chips to the grill (if using).

2. Brush the ribs all over with the hot sauce and then season with the salt, pepper, and garlic.

3. Place the ribs on the indirect side of the grill and close the lid. If using a charcoal grill, place the air vents above the ribs to direct the airflow over the meat.

4. Cook for 4 to 5 hours, adding more wood chips halfway through, until the internal temperature of the ribs reaches 210°F. (Try not to touch the bone with the thermometer when checking the temperature or you may get a false reading.)

5. Remove the ribs from the grill, cover loosely with aluminum foil, and let rest for 20 minutes before serving.

EZ BBQ TIP: If you don't want to babysit the grill for 4 hours (or more), finish these ribs in the oven. Add a second handful of wood chips when preheating the grill, to help infuse smoke into the meat more quickly, and cook for 1 hour at 325°F. Remove the ribs from the grill and finish cooking them in a 325°F oven for 3 to 4 hours, until their internal temperature reaches 210°F.

GRILLED BEEF FAJITA SALAD WITH CILANTRO-LIME DRESSING

DIRECT HEAT COOKING

SERVES 4 ★ **PREP TIME:** 10 MINUTES ★ **COOK TIME:** 20 MINUTES

TOOLS: Food processor, vegetable grill pan

This is a favorite dish for Sunday family dinners in our house as it is quick to make and on the healthier side. We like to grill all the vegetables in this recipe, including the romaine lettuce and the avocados. The sear on the lettuce completely changes the flavor of this dish, and the grilled avocados come out super creamy. I hope this dish becomes one of your family's favorites, too.

FOR THE DRESSING
2 bunches fresh cilantro
1 garlic clove, minced
¼ cup freshly squeezed lime juice
2 teaspoons honey
½ teaspoon ground cumin
½ teaspoon kosher salt
½ cup extra-virgin olive oil

FOR THE SALAD
2 tablespoons canola oil
1 pound skirt steak
2 teaspoons kosher salt, divided
2 teaspoons freshly ground black pepper, divided
2 romaine lettuce hearts, halved lengthwise
1 red, yellow, or orange bell pepper, cut into ½-inch strips
1 red onion, cut into ½-inch-wide strips
2 tablespoons olive oil
2 avocados, halved and pitted

1. In a food processor, combine the cilantro, garlic, lime juice, honey, cumin, salt, and olive oil. Pulse until smooth and creamy. Transfer the dressing to a serving container.

2. Preheat the grill to high heat (500°F) for direct heat cooking by lighting the heat source (or piling coals) in the spot that will be directly under the food. Put the canola oil on a folded paper towel and use a large pair of tongs to wipe down the grill grate with it.

3. Place the vegetable grill pan on one side of the grill to heat up.

4. Season the skirt steak with 1 teaspoon of salt and 1 teaspoon of pepper.

5. Lightly drizzle the romaine, bell pepper, and onion with 1½ tablespoons of olive oil. Rub the flesh side of the avocados with the remaining ½ tablespoon of olive oil. Season the vegetables with the remaining 1 teaspoon of salt and 1 teaspoon of pepper. Place the onion and bell pepper in the hot grill pan.

6. Place the skirt steak on the grill and sear for 4 to 5 minutes, until it starts to develop a char. Flip the steak, then stir the vegetables. Cook the steak for 4 to 5 minutes more, until a char forms on the steak or the internal temperature reaches 130°F. Remove the steak from the grill, cover loosely with aluminum foil, and let it rest.

7. Place the romaine and the avocado, cut-side down, directly on the grill. Cook for 5 minutes, or until grill marks appear. Remove the vegetables from the grill and the grill pan. Chop the romaine and avocado.

8. Slice the skirt steak thinly against the grain into strips. Use a tablespoon to scoop the avocado out of its skin, maintaining its shape, then slice it.

9. In a large bowl, toss together the romaine, avocado, bell pepper, and onion. Top the salad with the steak strips and serve with the dressing on the side.

REVERSE SEARED COWBOY STEAK WITH CHIMICHURRI SAUCE

TWO-ZONE INDIRECT HEAT COOKING
SERVES 2 ★ PREP TIME: 10 MINUTES ★ **COOK TIME:** 30 MINUTES
TOOLS: Hickory or mesquite wood chips (optional), food processor

In my opinion, nothing says grilling like a big ol' steak, and the rib eye is the epitome of grilled steaks. This recipe uses a cowboy or tomahawk bone-in rib eye, which is typically 2 to 3 inches thick and can easily feed two people. The tomahawk steak includes the entire rib bone, which extends up to 12 inches, while the cowboy steak has a shorter rib bone, which extends about 3 inches. Keep the size of your grill in mind when shopping; make sure the steak you buy will fit! The chimichurri sauce is a variation of an Argentinean recipe, using both parsley and cilantro, and it gets just a little heat from a Fresno chile.

FOR THE STEAK
1 cowboy or tomahawk cut rib-eye steak
Kosher salt
Freshly ground black pepper

FOR THE CHIMICHURRI SAUCE
1 cup fresh Italian parsley leaves
1 cup fresh cilantro leaves
2 tablespoons coarsely chopped red onion
1 Fresno chile, seeded
4 to 6 garlic cloves, peeled
2 tablespoons red wine vinegar
1 tablespoon freshly squeezed lime juice
1½ teaspoons kosher salt
¾ cup extra-virgin olive oil

1. Preheat the grill to medium heat (350°F) for two-zone indirect heat cooking by lighting the heat source (or piling coals) on one side of the grill. Add a handful of hickory or mesquite wood chips to the grill (if using).

2. Season the steak with salt and pepper and place it on the indirect heat side of the grill. Monitor the steak and remove it from the grill after 20 to 22 minutes, or when it reaches 115°F, flipping it once halfway through cooking.

3. Increase the temperature of the grill to high heat (500°F).

4. While the steak cooks, in a food processor, combine the parsley, cilantro, onion, chile, garlic, vinegar, lime juice, and salt. Pulse until slightly chunky. Transfer the chimichurri to a small bowl and stir in the olive oil until fully incorporated. (Adding the olive oil last prevents the sauce from being fully pureed and preserves the texture of the ingredients.)

5. Once the grill reaches temperature, sear the steak for about 4 minutes per side, or until it reaches an internal temperature of 130°F. Remove the steak from the grill and let rest for 15 minutes.

6. Using a large chef's knife, carefully slice the rib eye from the bone. Cutting it against the grain, slice the rib eye into ½-inch strips. Drizzle the steak with the chimichurri sauce and serve.

EZ BBQ TIP: Remove the steak from the refrigerator before lighting the grill to let it get closer to room temperature. This will prevent the outside of the steak from cooking faster than the center.

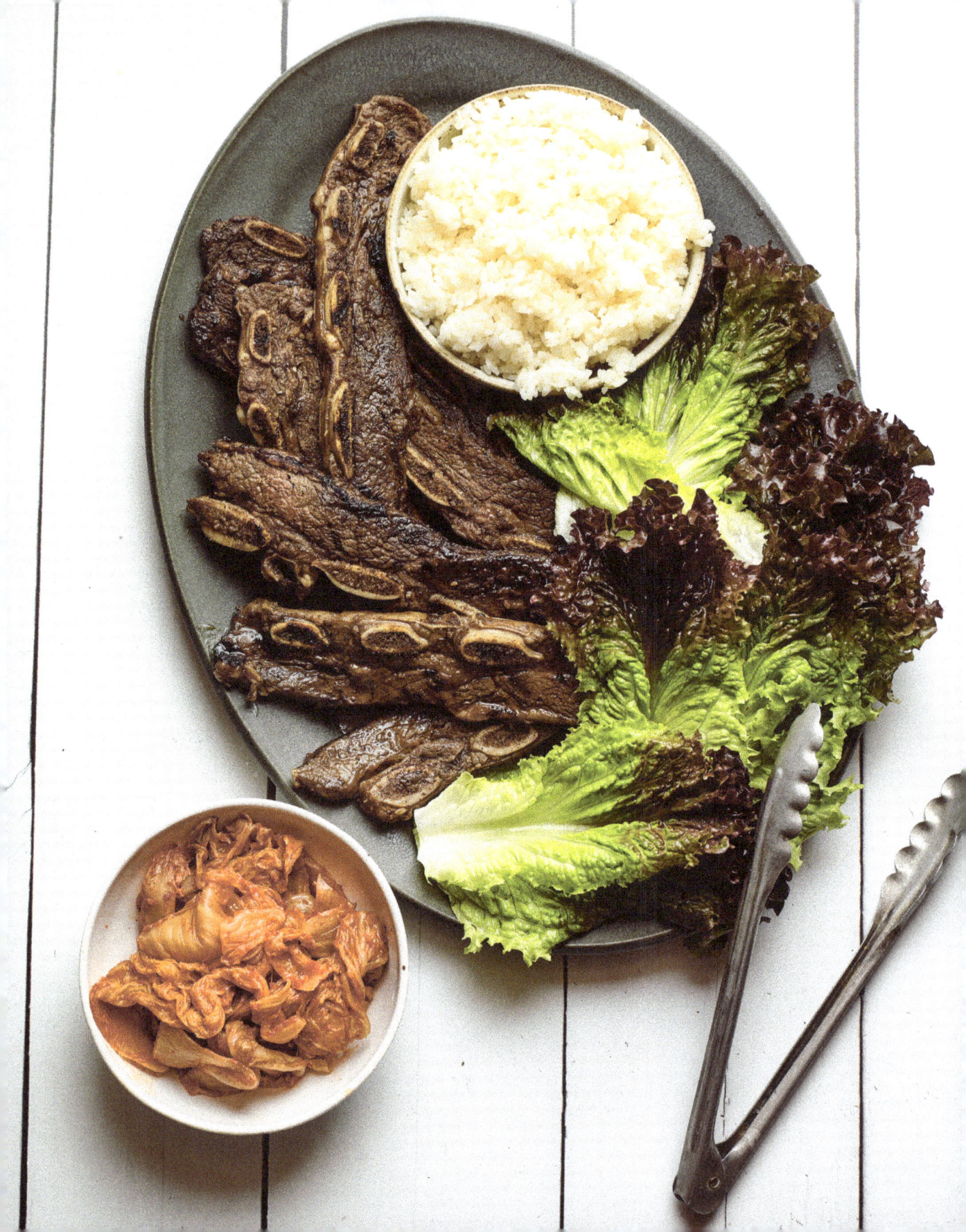

KOREAN-STYLE SHORT RIBS

DIRECT HEAT COOKING
SERVES 4 ★ **PREP TIME:** 5 MINUTES ★ **COOK TIME:** 10 MINUTES

Korean-style short ribs, also known as kalbi, are strips of beef cut across the rib bones. Look for Korean short ribs (also called flanken-style ribs) or have a butcher cut them for you. Korean ribs are often flavored with gochujang, a chile paste made from fermented soybeans mixed with red peppers, salt, and sugar that has a vinegary, spicy flavor. Look for a bright-red container in the Asian ingredients section of your grocery store or head to an Asian market to choose from a number of options. To turn these ribs into a traditional meal, serve the meat on lettuce leaves (green or red leaf) with cooked short-grain white rice and kimchi.

FOR THE MARINADE
3 tablespoons dark brown sugar
¼ cup peanut oil
3 garlic cloves, minced
3 tablespoons low-sodium soy sauce
1 teaspoon sesame oil
1 teaspoon ground ginger
1 tablespoon gochujang or red chili paste (optional)
3 pounds flanken-cut beef short ribs
2 tablespoons canola oil

1. In a gallon-size zip-top bag, combine the brown sugar, peanut oil, garlic, soy sauce, sesame oil, ginger, and gochujang (if using). Add the short ribs and seal the bag while pressing out any air. Massage the marinade thoroughly over the ribs.

2. Preheat the grill to high heat (500°F) for direct heat cooking by lighting the heat source (or piling coals) in the spot that will be directly under the food. Put the canola oil on a folded paper towel and use a large pair of tongs to wipe down the grill grate with it.

3. Remove the ribs from the marinade, discard the marinade, and place them on the grill. Cook for 3 to 4 minutes per side. (Note that flareups caused by the oil and sugar can occur; to avoid this from happening, when flipping the ribs, place them on a clean portion of the grill.)

4. Serve as whole strips or cut between the ribs for finger food–size servings.

GRILLED AL PASTOR SKEWERS

DIRECT HEAT COOKING
MAKES 10 SKEWERS ★ **PREP TIME:** 15 MINUTES + UP TO 3 DAYS TO MARINATE ★ **COOK TIME:** 20 MINUTES
TOOLS: 10 wooden skewers (soaked in water for at least 1 hour)

Al pastor was created in the early 20th century in Mexico when Lebanese immigrants combined their traditional vertical grilling techniques with local flavors and ingredients. It is based on a classic shawarma, but al pastor uses pork instead of lamb, and the spit is topped with pineapple instead of onion. My variation (which doesn't require a spit) can be marinated for up to 3 days but takes only 20 minutes to grill. The dish's base flavor and signature orange color come from achiote paste (see page 62).

FOR THE MARINADE
½ cup chicken stock
¼ cup white vinegar
1 (3.5-ounce) package achiote paste
2 teaspoons canola oil
2 teaspoons sugar
2 teaspoons kosher salt
1 teaspoon ground cumin
1 teaspoon dried oregano
1 teaspoon granulated garlic
Juice from 1 (16-ounce) can pineapple chunks

FOR THE SKEWERS
2 pounds pork shoulder or pork butt, cut into 1-inch cubes
2 tablespoons canola oil
1 (16-ounce) can pineapple chunks, including the juice
Lime wedges, for serving (optional)

1. In a gallon-size zip-top bag, combine the stock, vinegar, achiote paste, oil, sugar, salt, cumin, oregano, garlic, and pineapple juice. Seal the bag while pressing out any air and massage the bag until everything is well mixed.

2. Add the pork to the bag, seal the bag while pressing out any air, and massage the bag so the marinade covers the pork. Refrigerate the meat to marinate for up to 3 days, or at least 4 hours.

3. Preheat the grill to high heat (or 500°F) for direct heat cooking by lighting the heat source (or piling coals) in the spot that will be directly under the food. Put the oil on a folded paper towel and use a large pair of tongs to wipe down the grill grate with it.

4. Remove the meat from the marinade (discard the marinade), and thread 1 piece of pork onto a skewer followed by 1 pineapple chunk. Continue alternating pieces of pork and pineapple on the skewer, keeping the pork and pineapple closely packed together but leaving about 2 inches on one end of the skewer as a handle. Repeat the process with the remaining skewers.

5. Place the skewers on the grill and cook for 5 minutes per side, for a total of 20 minutes, or until the internal temperature of the pork reaches 145°F.

6. Remove the skewers from the grill, cover loosely with aluminum foil, and let rest for 5 minutes. Serve immediately with the lime wedges (if using).

SERVING SUGGESTION: Serve the cooked pork taco style on corn tortillas along with diced onion and fresh cilantro, topped with salsa verde. Squeeze some lime juice on top to add a bit of acid and balance the flavors.

MAPLE-BOURBON PORK CHOPS WITH SMOKED APPLESAUCE

TWO-ZONE INDIRECT HEAT COOKING + STOVETOP
SERVES 4 ★ PREP TIME: 15 MINUTES ★ **COOK TIME:** 42 MINUTES
TOOLS: Apple or hickory wood chips

The flavors in maple syrup and bourbon complement each other well, and the combination of ingredients helps form a nice crust on these grilled pork chops due to their sugar content. In this recipe, I pair the pork chops with applesauce that is flavored with smoke from the grill. When choosing your applesauce, look for a chunky variety with no sugar added as you will be providing the flavors.

FOR THE APPLESAUCE
- 1 (48-ounce) jar chunky no-sugar-added applesauce
- 1 teaspoon ground cinnamon
- 2 teaspoons dark brown sugar
- 1 teaspoon freshly squeezed lemon juice (optional)

FOR THE PORK CHOPS
- 4 (5-ounce) pork loin chops (about 1 inch thick)
- Canola oil
- 2 teaspoons kosher salt
- 2 teaspoons freshly ground black pepper
- 2 tablespoons unsalted butter, at room temperature
- 3 tablespoons maple syrup
- ⅓ cup bourbon

1. Preheat the grill to medium heat (350°F) for two-zone indirect heat cooking by lighting the heat source (or piling coals) on one side of the grill. Add a handful of apple or hickory wood chips to the grill.

2. In a disposable aluminum pan, stir together the applesauce, cinnamon, brown sugar, and lemon juice (if using). Place the pan on the indirect side of the grill, close the lid, and smoke for 20 minutes.

3. Meanwhile, pat the pork chops dry with a paper towel and lightly coat them with oil. Season the meat with salt and pepper.

4. In a small saucepan on the stovetop over medium-low heat, melt the butter and maple syrup. Carefully stir in the bourbon, turn the heat to medium, and cook the glaze for 10 minutes, or until it starts to reduce and thicken. Remove from the heat.

5. Remove the applesauce from the grill. Add more wood chips to the grill and let them heat until they produce white smoke.

6. Place the pork chops on the indirect heat side of the grill, close the lid, and let the chops smoke for 10 minutes.

7. Move the chops to the direct heat side of the grill and brush the tops of the chops with the maple-bourbon sauce. Cook for 2 minutes, flip the chops, and glaze them. Continue this process, flipping and glazing every 2 minutes, for 4 to 6 minutes, or until the internal temperature of the pork reaches 145°F.

8. Remove the pork chops from the grill, cover loosely with aluminum foil, and let them rest for 5 minutes. Serve with the smoked applesauce and remaining maple-bourbon sauce on the side.

CHAR SIU PORK TENDERLOIN

DIRECT HEAT COOKING

SERVES 4 ★ PREP TIME: 10 MINUTES + 4 HOURS TO MARINATE, OR OVERNIGHT
COOK TIME: 25 MINUTES

Char siu is a type of Cantonese-style roasted pork that has a sweet and salty flavor. This dish can be made with various cuts of pork, but I have chosen pork tenderloin, a cut found along the pig's backbone that is known for its flavor and tenderness. The pork can be prepared in advance and marinated overnight. The red food coloring is optional but gives the pork its traditional red hue.

2 (1¼-pound) pork tenderloins

FOR THE MARINADE
½ cup teriyaki sauce
¼ cup chicken stock
¼ cup ketchup
¼ cup soy sauce
2 tablespoons hoisin sauce
2 tablespoons Shaoxing (Chinese cooking) wine
4 garlic cloves, minced
2 teaspoons Chinese five-spice powder
4 drops red food coloring (optional)
2 tablespoons canola oil

1. Trim the tenderloins of any excess fat or silver skin (the thin, fibrous membrane on the meat).

2. In a small bowl, whisk the teriyaki sauce, stock, ketchup, soy sauce, hoisin, wine, garlic, five-spice powder, and food coloring (if using) well. Set aside ¼ cup of the sauce to use during grilling and pour the rest into a gallon-size zip-top bag.

3. Place the pork tenderloins in the bag and seal the bag, pressing out any air. Massage the bag so the marinade covers the pork. Refrigerate overnight, if possible, or for at least 4 hours.

4. Preheat the grill to medium-high heat (450°F) for direct heat cooking by lighting the heat source (or piling coals) in the spot that will be directly under the food. Put the oil on a folded paper towel and use a large pair of tongs to wipe down the grill grate with it.

5. Remove the pork from the marinade (discard the marinade), place the meat on the grill, and close the lid. Cook for about 25 minutes, flipping the meat a quarter turn and basting it with the reserved sauce every 5 minutes, to grill all four sides, or until the pork reaches an internal temperature of 140°F.

6. Remove the pork from the grill, cover loosely with aluminum foil, and let rest for 5 minutes.

7. Slice the pork into ½-inch pieces to serve.

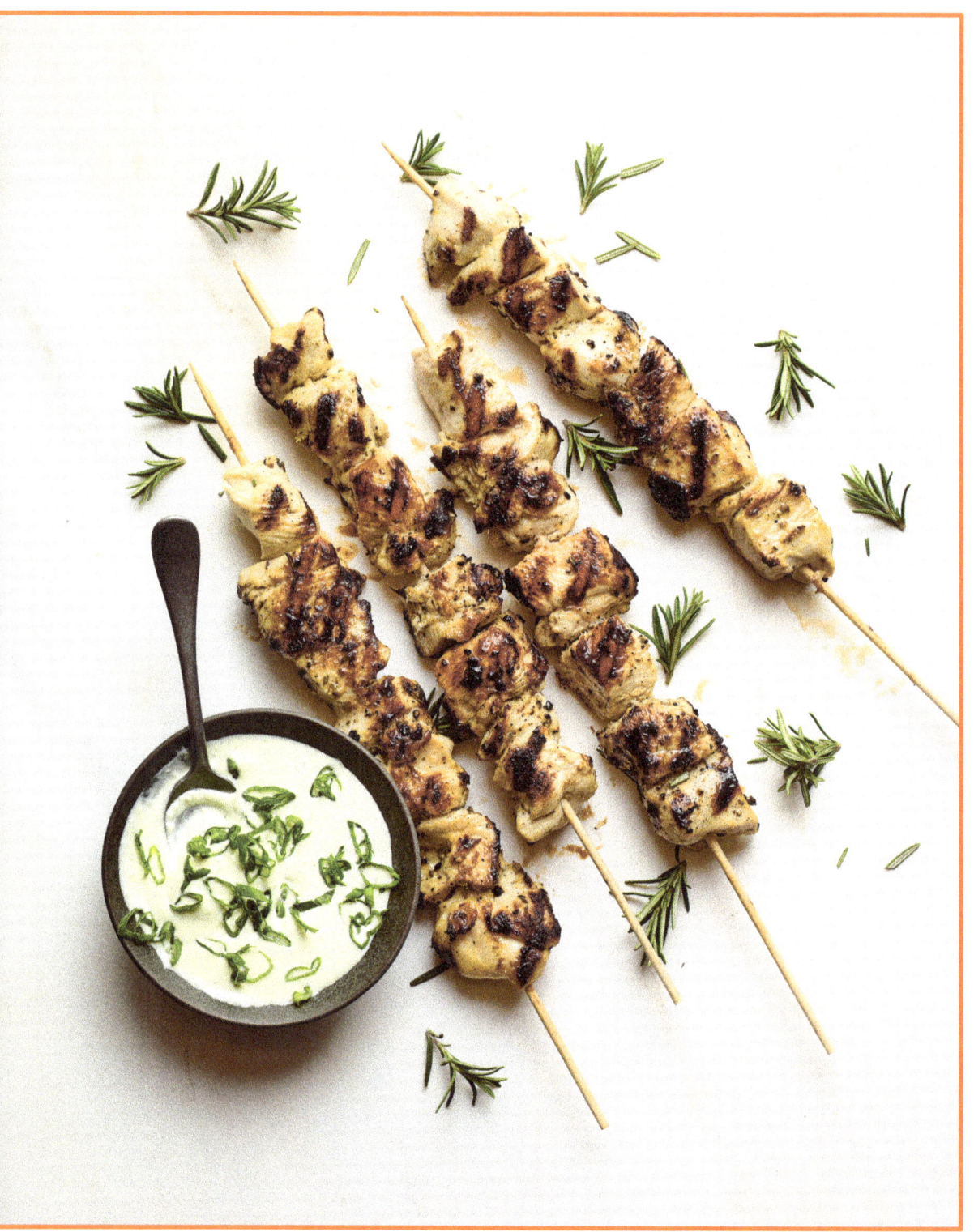

CHAPTER 4

POULTRY

SPICY KOREAN-STYLE CHICKEN **52**

CITRUS-MARINATED CHICKEN **54**

GRILLED CHICKEN TINGA **55**

GRILLED HULI HULI–STYLE CHICKEN **57**

★ LEMON-DIJON-ROSEMARY SKEWERS **58** ★

MAPLE-DIJON GRILLED CHICKEN **60**

GRILLED NASHVILLE HOT CHICKEN **61**

POLLO AL CARBON **62**

CENTRAL TEXAS–STYLE BBQ TURKEY BREAST **64**

CHARCOAL CHIMNEY YAKITORI CHICKEN **66**

POULTRY CHEAT SHEET

BBQ COOKING STYLES

Direct heat:
350° to 450°F, medium heat, for boneless and skinless poultry
Two-zone indirect heat:
350° to 450°F, medium heat, for bone-in poultry

INTERNAL TEMPS

FOOD TYPE	INTERNAL TEMPS
Chicken and turkey breasts	165°F for safe consumption
Chicken and turkey bone-in thighs and legs	175°F for safe consumption
Duck breasts	135°F to 140°F to avoid drying out the meat
Duck bone-in thighs and legs	165°F to break down the connective tissue

USEFUL TOOLS

Large zip-top bags: Although they may seem low-tech, gallon-size zip-top bags are quite useful for preparing poultry. You can use them to maximize the marinating process (most chicken dishes call for marination) by concentrating the liquid around the meat. And they are handy for tenderizing meat: Put the raw meat into a bag before you hit it with your mallet and the meat juices won't go splattering around your workstation.

KEEP IN MIND

High Sodium: Most poultry sold in grocery stores today can contain upward of 30 percent saline solution because of the process of "plumping." For the same reason, a serving of poultry can contain 500 mg or more of sodium. When shopping for your bird, read the label on the package and find one with the lowest percentage of solution or brine. You should also hold back a little on the salt when seasoning poultry and add more to taste once the dish is completed.

COMMON PROBLEMS

Uneven Cooking: A common problem when grilling poultry is cooking it at too high of a temperature. Bone-in meat should be cooked at lower temperatures, allowing the heat to slowly penetrate the meat, so it cooks evenly. At higher temperatures, the outside of the bird will overcook and lose moisture while the inside is still underdone.

ALSO TRY

Air Drying: If you are having a hard time getting crispy skin on your poultry (a problem often created by the extra moisture from "plumping"), let the bird air-dry, uncovered, in the refrigerator for up to two days, then add a light coat of oil to the skin before cooking. This process will dry out the skin using the dry air in your refrigerator and the oil will assist in the quicker transfer of heat. I've even heard of some cooks using a hair dryer to speed up this process.

SPICY KOREAN-STYLE CHICKEN

DIRECT HEAT COOKING
SERVES 4 ★ **PREP TIME:** 10 MINUTES + 1 TO 4 HOURS TO MARINATE ★ **COOK TIME:** 15 MINUTES

This recipe is an adaptation of the wildly popular Korean fried chicken but made for the barbecue instead of the deep fryer. The chicken is smothered in gochujang chile sauce, which is made from fermented soybeans mixed with red peppers, salt, and sugar. It has a wonderful spicy, vinegary flavor.

FOR THE SAUCE
¼ cup canola oil, plus 2 tablespoons
¼ cup gochujang
2 tablespoons toasted sesame oil
¼ cup low-sodium soy sauce
3 tablespoons light brown sugar
4 teaspoons ground ginger
2 tablespoons minced garlic
2 teaspoons kosher salt
1 teaspoon ground white pepper
2 pounds boneless, skinless chicken thighs

1. In a small bowl, stir together ¼ cup of canola oil, the gochujang, sesame oil, soy sauce, brown sugar, ginger, garlic, salt, and pepper.

2. Trim the chicken of any excess fat, then place the chicken in a gallon-size zip-top bag. Pour half of the gochujang sauce into the bag and seal it while pressing out any air. Massage the sauce over the chicken and refrigerate it for at least 1 hour and preferably 4. Refrigerate the remaining sauce in an airtight container.

3. Preheat the grill to medium-high heat (450°F) for direct heat cooking by lighting the heat source (or piling coals) in the spot that will be directly under the food. Put the remaining 2 tablespoons of canola oil on a folded paper towel and use a large pair of tongs to wipe down the grill grate with it.

4. Let the chicken and reserved sauce come to room temperature while the grill preheats.

5. Remove the chicken from the zip-top bag, discard the marinade in the bag, and place the chicken on the grill, smooth-side down. Brush the side of the chicken facing up with some of the reserved sauce and grill the chicken for 7 minutes. Flip the chicken, brush it with more sauce, and cook it for 7 minutes more. The chicken is done when the internal temperature reaches 165°F. Remove the chicken from the grill and cover loosely with aluminum foil. Let the chicken rest for 10 minutes before serving it with the remaining sauce.

CITRUS-MARINATED CHICKEN

TWO-ZONE INDIRECT HEAT COOKING
SERVES 4 ★ PREP TIME: 10 MINUTES + 2 TO 8 HOURS TO MARINATE ★ **COOK TIME:** 30 MINUTES

Inspired by one of our favorite chicken places in Southern California, this dish features the flavors of oranges, pineapples, and lime. The chicken is grilled directly over the heat to get a nice char and then finished on the indirect side of the grill.

8 bone-in, skin-on chicken thighs (about 2½ pounds)

FOR THE MARINADE
1 cup pineapple juice
¼ cup orange juice
2 tablespoons freshly squeezed lime juice
2 tablespoons light brown sugar
1 tablespoon kosher salt
1 tablespoon white vinegar
2 teaspoons chili powder
1 teaspoon dried oregano
½ teaspoon freshly ground black pepper
½ teaspoon cayenne pepper
1 teaspoon granulated garlic

2 tablespoons canola oil

1. Place the chicken thighs in a gallon-size zip-top bag and pour in the pineapple, orange, and lime juices. Add the brown sugar, salt, vinegar, chili powder, oregano, black pepper, cayenne, and garlic. Seal the bag while pressing out any air. Massage the marinade over the chicken and refrigerate it for at least 2 hours.

2. Preheat the grill to medium-high heat (425°F) for two-zone indirect cooking by lighting the heat source (or piling coals) on one side of the grill. Put the oil on a folded paper towel and use a large pair of tongs to wipe down the grill grate.

3. Remove the chicken from the marinade and place it, skin-side down, on the direct heat side of the grill. Discard the marinade. Cook the chicken for 7 minutes, then flip it and grill it for 7 minutes more.

4. Transfer the chicken to the indirect side of the grill, skin-side up, and cook it for 10 to 12 minutes, or until the internal temperature reaches 175°F. Remove the chicken from the grill, cover loosely with aluminum foil, and let the chicken rest for 5 minutes before serving.

GRILLED CHICKEN TINGA

TWO-ZONE INDIRECT HEAT COOKING
SERVES 4 ★ PREP TIME: 10 MINUTES + 30 MINUTES TO MARINATE ★ **COOK TIME:** 1 HOUR
TOOLS: Food processor

My son Kenny used to be a chef in Denver, and one of the best things he would make for us was chicken tinga. An all-day, slow-cooked dish, tinga is flavored with chipotle peppers in adobo sauce, tomatoes, and onions. This version is an adaptation of that recipe, but it is made for the grill and is cooked in an hour.

FOR THE MARINADE
1 (10-ounce) can fire-roasted tomatoes
1 (7-ounce) can chipotles in adobo sauce
½ medium sweet onion, coarsely chopped
4 garlic cloves, peeled
2 teaspoons dried oregano
2 teaspoons ground cumin
2 teaspoons kosher salt
2 teaspoons freshly ground black pepper
½ cup chicken stock

2 (2-pound) half chickens

1. In a food processor, pulse the tomatoes, chipotles with their sauce, onion, garlic, oregano, cumin, salt, pepper, and stock until the marinade is fully combined and smooth. Place the chicken halves into a gallon-size zip-top bag along with half the marinade. Seal the bag while pressing out any air. Massage the marinade over the chicken and refrigerate it for 30 minutes. Set aside the remaining marinade.

2. Preheat the grill to medium heat (350°F) for two-zone indirect heat cooking by lighting the heat source (or piling coals) on one side of the grill.

3. Remove the chicken from the zip-top bag and place it, skin-side down, on the direct heat side of the grill. Pour the marinade from the bag over the bone side of the chicken and spread it evenly. Close the lid and cook the chicken for 15 minutes. Flip the chicken over, close the lid, and cook for 15 minutes more.

4. Move the chicken to the indirect side of the grill, skin-side up, close the lid, and cook for 15 minutes. Pour the reserved marinade over the chicken, close the lid, and cook for 15 minutes, or until the chicken reaches an internal temperature of 165°F. Remove the chicken from the grill, cover loosely with aluminum foil, and let rest for 5 minutes before slicing and serving.

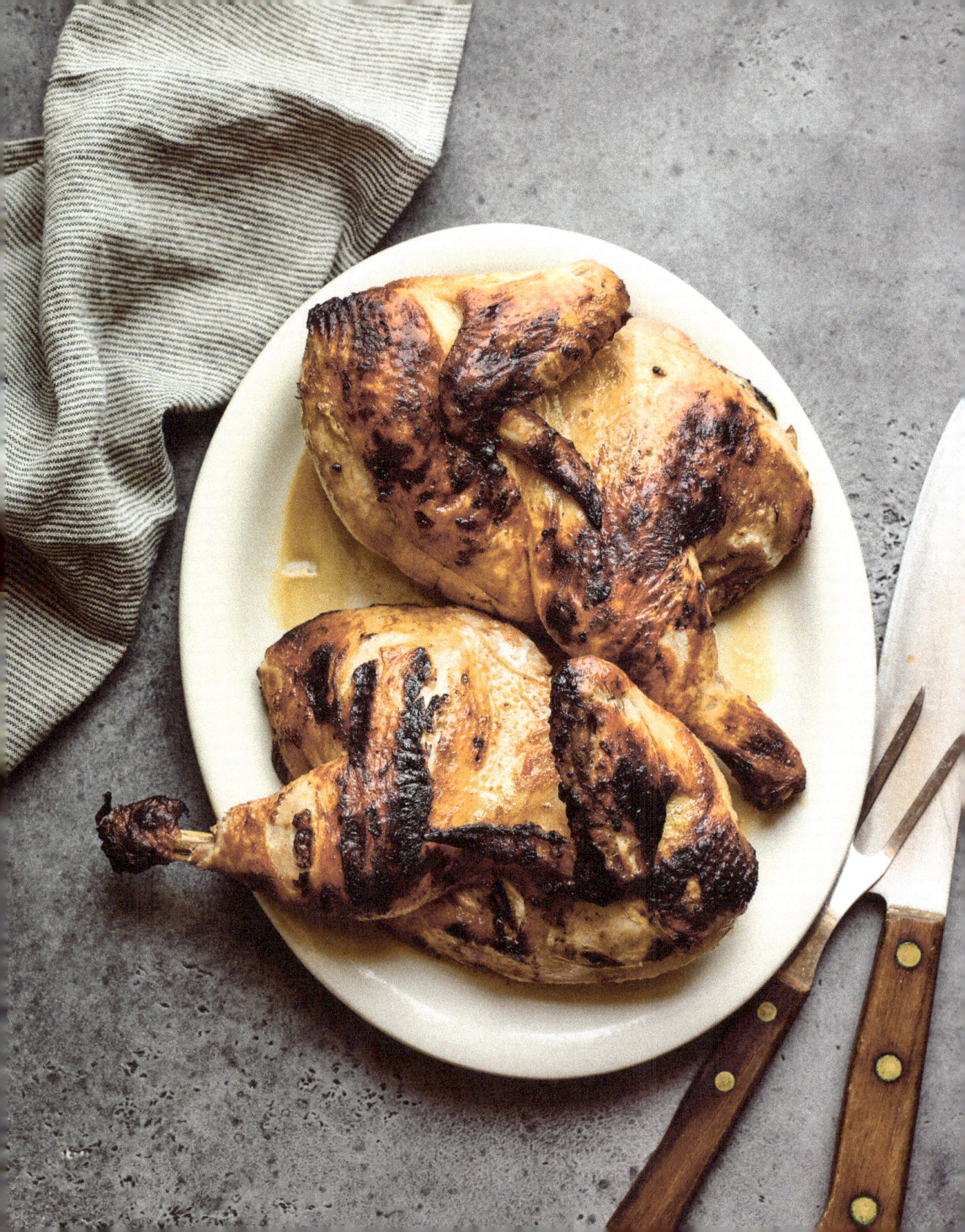

GRILLED HULI HULI-STYLE CHICKEN

DIRECT HEAT COOKING
SERVES 4 ★ **PREP TIME:** 10 MINUTES + 2 HOURS TO MARINATE ★ **COOK TIME:** 40 MINUTES
TOOLS: Mesquite wood chips

This chicken dish was made famous at roadside chicken stands in Hawaii in the 1950s. The word *huli* means "to turn" in Hawaiian and refers to the process of constantly turning the chicken on a rotisserie. Here, I flip the birds repeatedly. I have also added sriracha sauce, for just a bit of heat.

FOR THE MARINADE
1 cup pineapple juice
½ cup ketchup
¼ cup mirin (also sold as Aji-Mirin)
3 tablespoons light brown sugar
2 tablespoons rice vinegar
4 garlic cloves, minced
1 tablespoon toasted sesame oil
1 tablespoon sriracha
1 teaspoon powdered ginger

2 (1½-pound) half chickens
2 tablespoons canola oil

1. In a small bowl, stir together the pineapple juice, ketchup, mirin, brown sugar, vinegar, garlic, sesame oil, sriracha, and ginger to make a marinade. Set aside ¾ cup of marinade in the refrigerator for basting.

2. Place the chickens and the remaining marinade in a gallon-size zip-top bag and seal the bag while pressing out any air. Massage the marinade over the chickens and refrigerate for at least 2 hours and up to 24 hours.

3. Preheat the grill to medium-high heat (400°F) for direct heat cooking by lighting the heat source (or piling coals) in the spot that will be directly under the food. Add a handful of mesquite wood chips to the grill. Put the canola oil on a folded paper towel and use a large pair of tongs to wipe down the grill grate with it.

4. Place the chickens on the grill, skin-side down, and baste liberally with the reserved marinade. Cook the chickens for 5 minutes. Flip them, baste again, and cook for 5 minutes more. Continue flipping and basting the chickens every 5 minutes for 35 to 40 minutes, until the internal temperature reaches 165°F.

5. Remove the chicken from the grill, cover loosely with aluminum foil, and let sit for 10 minutes before serving.

LEMON-DIJON-ROSEMARY SKEWERS

DIRECT HEAT COOKING
MAKES 4 SKEWERS ★ PREP TIME: 15 MINUTES ★ **COOK TIME:** 12 MINUTES
TOOLS: 4 wooden skewers (soaked in water for at least 1 hour), food processor

This dish is quick and easy to make and includes a Greek-inspired feta cheese and yogurt dipping sauce. The flavors are inspired by the Mediterranean region: Dijon mustard hails from the central part of France; olive oil comes from Spain and Italy; rosemary is prevalent along the coastal region of the Mediterranean Sea; and feta cheese originated in the Greek islands.

1 pound boneless, skinless chicken breasts, cut into 2-inch cubes
1 tablespoon Dijon mustard
1 tablespoon extra-virgin olive oil
Juice of ½ lemon
Grated zest of ½ lemon
1 teaspoon kosher salt

1 teaspoon freshly ground black pepper
3 garlic cloves, minced
1 teaspoon fresh rosemary leaves, coarsely chopped
2 tablespoons canola oil

FOR THE DIPPING SAUCE
4 ounces feta cheese
1 cup plain yogurt

3 tablespoons fresh parsley, coarsely chopped
2 tablespoons coarsely chopped scallions, white and green parts
1 garlic clove, minced
Juice of ½ lemon
Grated zest of ½ lemon

1. In a gallon-size zip-top bag, combine the chicken, mustard, olive oil, lemon juice, lemon zest, salt, pepper, garlic, and rosemary. Seal the bag while pressing out any air. Thoroughly massage the mustard mixture all over the chicken, then refrigerate to marinate.

2. Preheat the grill to medium heat (350°) for direct heat cooking by lighting the heat source (or piling coals) in the spot that will be directly under the food. Put the canola oil on a folded paper towel and use a large pair of tongs to wipe down the grill grate with it.

3. In a food processor, pulse together the feta, yogurt, parsley, scallions, garlic, lemon juice, and lemon zest until fully incorporated. Transfer the sauce to a small bowl.

4. Thread 4 or 5 pieces of marinated chicken onto each skewer. Place them on the grill and cook for 4 to 6 minutes per side, until the chicken reaches an internal temperature of 165°F. Remove the skewers from the grill, cover loosely with aluminum foil, and let them rest for 10 minutes.

5. Serve with the feta dipping sauce on the side.

MAPLE-DIJON GRILLED CHICKEN

DIRECT HEAT COOKING
SERVES 4 ★ PREP TIME: 15 MINUTES ★ **COOK TIME:** 16 MINUTES
TOOLS: Meat mallet or tenderizer with a flat surface

This quick and easy dish features maple syrup and mustard. To get the best flavor out of this combination, use "grade B" maple syrup (also called "grade A very dark"), which has a bolder maple flavor than the stuff you have on hand for pancakes. This recipe also asks you to pound out the chicken breasts to create a uniform thickness, which allows for a more even cook.

- 4 (6-ounce) boneless, skinless chicken breasts
- ½ cup maple syrup
- ⅓ cup course-ground Dijon mustard
- 3 garlic cloves, minced
- 2 tablespoons canola oil

1. Working with one chicken breast at a time, place it inside a gallon-size zip-top bag and seal the bag while pressing out any air. Using the flat side of a meat mallet or tenderizer, gently pound the chicken until it is completely flat and roughly ½ inch thick. Remove the chicken breast from the bag and repeat the process with the remaining breasts, then return them all to the zip-top bag. (If the bag has any holes in it, use a new bag for this step.)

2. In a small bowl, whisk together the maple syrup, mustard, and garlic. Pour half the maple syrup mixture into the bag with the chicken and seal the bag while pressing out any air. Thoroughly massage the mixture onto the chicken.

3. Preheat the grill to medium-high heat (400°F) for direct heat cooking by lighting the heat source (or piling coals) in the spot that will be directly under the food. Put the oil on a folded paper towel and use a large pair of tongs to wipe down the grill grate with it.

4. Place the chicken on the grill and cook it for 7 to 8 minutes. Flip the chicken and cook for 7 to 8 minutes more, until it reaches an internal temperature of 165°F.

5. Remove the chicken from the grill, cover loosely with aluminum foil, and let it rest for 5 minutes. Slice the chicken before serving.

EZ BBQ TIP: If you do not have a meat mallet, a cast-iron skillet or a heavy saucepan will work just as well.

GRILLED NASHVILLE HOT CHICKEN

DIRECT HEAT COOKING
SERVES 4 ★ **PREP TIME:** 10 MINUTES + 4 TO 12 HOURS TO MARINATE ★ **COOK TIME:** 30 MINUTES

According to Nashville lore, this dish was created by a woman who sought revenge on her womanizing boyfriend by making him extremely spicy fried chicken. Instead of hating the spiciness, the boyfriend loved the dish so much that he and his brothers started a chicken shack. I have adapted this fiery dish for the grill and added a twist by marinating the chicken in pickle juice.

- 8 bone-in chicken thighs (about 2½ pounds)
- 1 (16-ounce) jar dill pickle slices, brine and pickles separated
- ¾ cup canola oil, plus 2 tablespoons
- ⅓ cup cayenne pepper
- 1½ tablespoons light brown sugar
- 1½ tablespoons smoked paprika
- 1 tablespoon chili powder
- 1 teaspoon granulated garlic
- 2 teaspoons kosher salt

1. In a gallon-size zip-top bag, combine the chicken and pickle brine. Seal the bag while pressing out any air. Refrigerate to marinate for at least 4 hours and up to 12 hours. Flip the bag over occasionally to make sure all parts of the chicken get soaked in brine. In a small bowl, stir together ¾ cup of oil, the cayenne, brown sugar, paprika, chili powder, garlic, and salt.

2. Preheat the grill to medium-high heat (400°F) for direct heat cooking by lighting the heat source (or piling coals) in the spot that will be directly under the food. Put the remaining 2 tablespoons of oil on a folded paper towel and use a large pair of tongs to wipe down the grill grate with it.

3. While the grill preheats, drain the pickle juice from the zip-top bag. Spoon the spice mixture into the bag and reseal the bag while pressing out any air. Vigorously massage the spice mixture onto the chicken.

4. Place the chicken on the grill, skin-side down. Cook for 10 minutes, flip the chicken, and cook it for 15 to 20 minutes, until it reaches an internal temperature of 175°F.

5. Remove the chicken from the grill, cover loosely with aluminum foil, and let it rest for 10 minutes. Serve the hot chicken with pickle slices on the side.

POLLO AL CARBON

DIRECT HEAT COOKING
SERVES 4 ★ PREP TIME: 10 MINUTES + 1 TO 4 HOURS
TO MARINATE ★ **COOK TIME:** 14 MINUTES
TOOLS: Mesquite or hickory wood chips, blender

This Tex-Mex favorite features achiote paste, which is a slightly spicy, smoky spice made of annatto seeds, cloves, coriander, cumin, garlic, and Mexican oregano. It can typically be found in 3.5-ounce packages in the Mexican sections of larger grocery stores or in Mexican markets, and it is readily available online. I also add a bit of non-traditional soy sauce to my recipe, as it brings a savory flavor that is hard to replicate with other ingredients. The chicken is grilled fairly hot and fast, and it will have some char on it when done, which adds even more flavor to this dish.

FOR THE MARINADE
- 1 cup pulp-free orange juice
- Juice of 1 lime
- Grated zest of 1 lime
- 1 (3.5-ounce) packet achiote paste
- 2 tablespoons chili powder
- 1½ tablespoons soy sauce
- 1 tablespoon kosher salt
- 2 teaspoons dried oregano
- 1 teaspoon ground cumin
- 2 tablespoons canola oil
- 8 boneless chicken thighs (about 2 pounds)
- 2 tablespoons canola oil

1. In a blender, combine the orange juice, lime juice, lime zest, achiote paste, chili powder, soy sauce, salt, oregano, cumin, and oil. Blend the marinade until smooth.

2. In a gallon-size zip-top bag, combine the chicken and 1 cup of marinade. Seal the bag while pressing out any air. Massage the marinade onto the chicken, making sure it is fully coated. Refrigerate for at least 1 hour and up to 4 hours. Reserve the remaining marinade.

3. Preheat the grill to medium-high heat (450°F) for direct heat cooking by lighting the heat source (or piling coals) in the spot that will be directly under the food. Add a handful of mesquite or hickory wood chips to the grill. Put the oil on a folded paper towel and use a large pair of tongs to wipe down the grill grate with it.

4. While the grill preheats, remove the chicken from the refrigerator and let it come to room temperature.

5. Place the chicken on the grill, skin-side down. Discard the marinade in the bag. Brush the side of the chicken facing up with some of the reserved marinade. Grill the chicken for 7 minutes, then flip it, brush the chicken with more marinade, and cook it for 7 minutes more, until it reaches an internal temperature of 165°F. Remove the chicken from the grill, cover loosely with aluminum foil, and let it rest for 5 minutes before serving.

EZ BBQ TIP: This recipe (like many others in the book) has you cook meats skin-side down first, which serves two purposes: First, you should always cook the presentation side down first. The presentation side is the side of the dish that faces up toward the diner. Remember, you eat with your eyes first. Second, when cooking poultry it allows a good sear on the skin, helping it to tighten up and lose its rubbery texture.

CENTRAL TEXAS-STYLE BBQ TURKEY BREAST

INDIRECT HEAT COOKING

SERVES 4 ★ **PREP TIME:** 5 MINUTES ★ **COOK TIME:** 1 HOUR

TOOLS: Hickory wood chips, heavy-duty aluminum foil

Our son Christian recently competed in the American Royal World Series of Barbecue in Kansas City, which is the largest barbecue competition in the world. He competed with a dish inspired by Central Texas–style turkey, which uses a simple application of a salt and pepper rub, affectionately known as Dalmatian Rub. My version of this turkey dish is black pepper forward and gets added flavor from hickory wood chips.

- 2 tablespoons canola oil
- 2 tablespoons freshly ground black pepper
- 4 teaspoons kosher salt
- 3 pounds boneless, skinless turkey breast
- 2 teaspoons mayonnaise
- 4 tablespoons (½ stick) cold unsalted butter, cut into 4 pieces

1. Preheat the grill to medium-high heat (400°F) for indirect heat cooking by lighting only the heat source (or piling coals) across from where you will place the food. Add a handful of hickory wood chips to your fire. Put the oil on a folded paper towel and use a large pair of tongs to wipe down the grill grate with it.

2. In a small bowl, stir together the pepper and salt. Rub the turkey breast with the mayonnaise (this acts as a binder) and season it generously with the pepper-salt mixture.

3. Place the turkey, skin-side down on the indirect heat side of the grill, close the lid, and cook for 20 minutes. Flip the turkey, close the lid, and cook the meat for 20 minutes more, until the internal temperature reaches 150°F.

4. Tear a piece of aluminum foil into an 18-by-18 inch square and place the butter pieces on the foil. Remove the turkey from the grill and place it on the butter. Wrap and seal the foil around the meat to make an airtight packet and put the packet on the indirect side of the grill for 10 minutes. Flip the foil packet and cook for 10 minutes more, until the meat's internal temperature reaches 165°F.

5. Remove the packet from the grill and let it rest for 10 minutes before carefully opening the foil. Slice the turkey and serve.

EZ BBQ TIP: When shopping for turkey breast, look for one that has not been pre-brined, so the flavor of the turkey shines. If your turkey breast comes in netting, do not remove it until after cooking, or the breast will fall apart.

CHARCOAL CHIMNEY YAKITORI CHICKEN

STOVETOP + DIRECT HEAT COOKING
MAKES 4 SKEWERS ★ **PREP TIME:** 15 MINUTES ★ **COOK TIME:** 31 MINUTES
TOOLS: Charcoal chimney, 50 briquettes, 8 metal skewers

My family and I lived in Southern California for seven years, and one of our favorite treats was to go into Los Angeles and have yakitori chicken in Little Tokyo. The chicken is grilled on skewers over a shallow, narrow grill called a *binchotan*. The meat is grilled inches away from the coals and is turned constantly to lightly char the meat but not burn it.

I replicate this cooking technique by keeping charcoal inside a chimney and cooking the meat directly over that, instead of putting the coals into the grill. I use standard charcoal briquettes for this recipe, but this would be a good time to experiment with binchotan charcoal (see page 10) to get a more authentic experience and flavor.

FOR THE SAUCE
- ⅔ cup low-sodium soy sauce
- ⅔ cup mirin (also sold as Aji-Mirin)
- ⅔ cup sake
- ⅔ cup water
- 3 tablespoons brown sugar
- 1 teaspoon freshly ground black pepper

FOR THE CHICKEN
- 2 pounds boneless, skinless chicken thighs, cut into 2-inch squares
- 4 scallions, white and green parts, cut into 1½-inch pieces
- Canola oil, for brushing the skewers
- 2 teaspoons kosher salt

1. In a small saucepan on the stovetop over medium-high heat, combine the soy sauce, mirin, sake, water, brown sugar, and pepper. Bring the sauce to a boil, then reduce the heat to low. Simmer for 10 to 15 minutes, or until the sauce thickens. The sauce is done when it coats the back of a spoon. Transfer the sauce to a small bowl or jar.

2. Fill a charcoal chimney halfway full, using about 50 briquettes, and light it.

3. When preparing the chicken for the grill, double up on the skewers (see tip). Fold a chicken thigh square in half and pierce it with the skewers. Pierce one of the scallion pieces, so it is parallel to the chicken. Repeat the process until you have 4 pieces of chicken and 3 scallions per skewer, arranging the chicken and scallions so they are centered on the skewers. Brush the chicken and scallions with oil and sprinkle with salt.

4. Once the charcoal has ashed over completely, after about 15 minutes, place 2 skewers across the opening of the chimney and brush some sauce onto the chicken. Every 2 minutes, flip the chicken skewers and brush them with sauce. Repeat the process until you have completed 4 flips. Remove from the grill and cover with aluminum foil. Repeat with the remaining skewers and sauce. Serve with any remaining sauce.

EZ BBQ TIP: I double up on the skewers for my yakitori, which helps keep the meat from spinning or falling off.

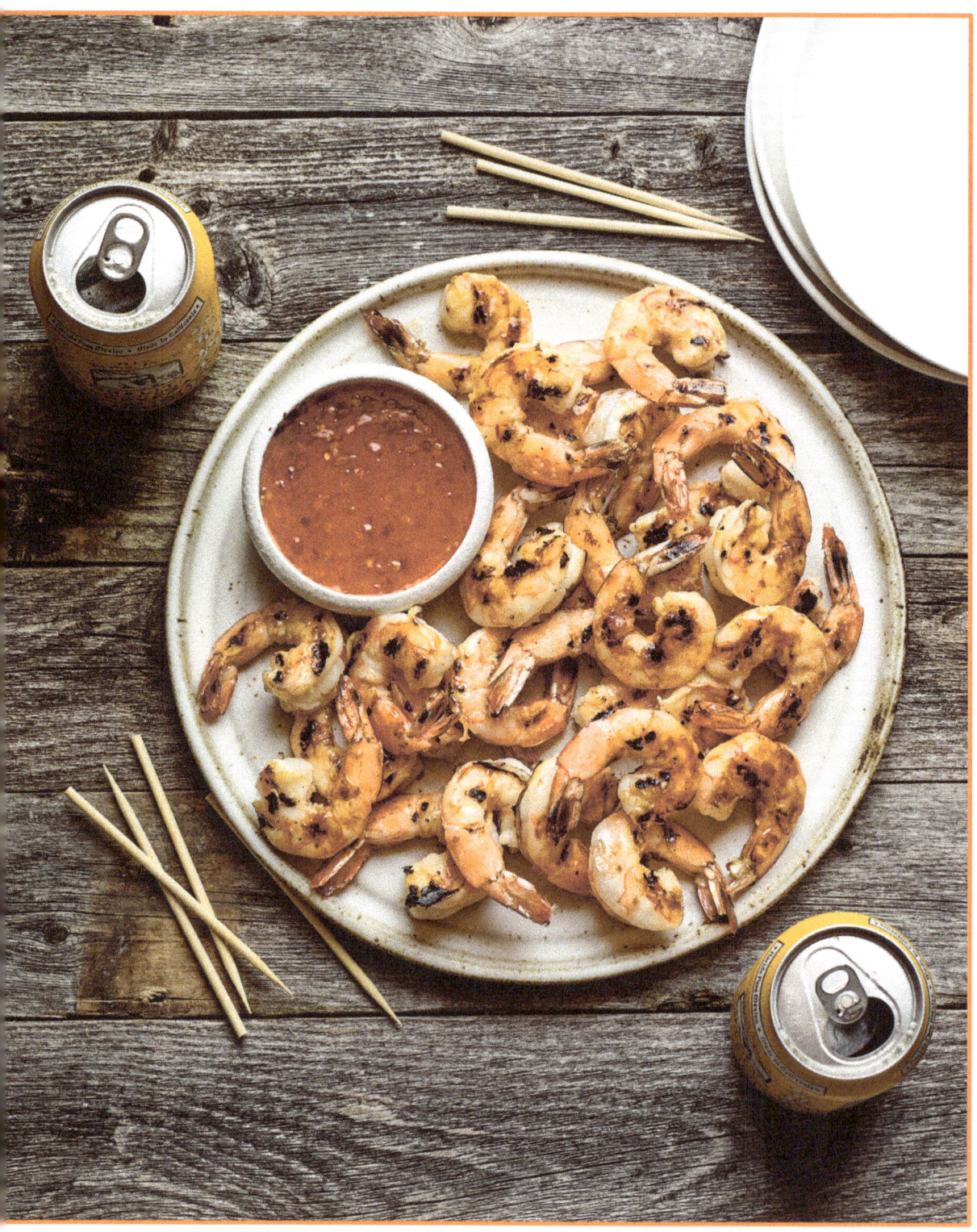

CHAPTER 5

SEAFOOD

★ SWEET CHILI SHRIMP 72 ★

FOIL PACKET SHRIMP "BOIL" 73

CAJUN BLACKENED GRILLED FISH 74

GRILLED SWORDFISH WITH RED PEPPER SAUCE 76

JAMAICAN JERK GRILLED HALIBUT 78

PARMESAN-CRUSTED GRILLED WHITEFISH 79

CEDAR PLANK TERIYAKI SALMON 81

TILAPIA PUTTANESCA 82

SEAFOOD CHEAT SHEET

Grilling seafood can sometimes be stressful for novice cooks, because it is delicate and can overcook or break easily. That said, all varieties of seafood can be grilled successfully.

BBQ COOKING STYLES

Direct heat:
350°F, medium heat
400°F to 450°F, medium-high heat
400°F to 500°F, high heat

INTERNAL TEMPS

FOOD TYPE	MED. RARE	MEDIUM	OVERCOOKED
Most Fish		Fully cooked 145°F (Most fish will start to flake easily when done)	
Tuna and Salmon	130°F	145°F	Above 145°F

USEFUL TOOLS

Heavy-duty aluminum foil: Really sturdy foil is a useful tool when cooking seafood. It can be turned into a packet or a makeshift tray to lock in the moisture of your seafood. It can also assist in keeping oils or butter from dripping onto the heat and causing flare-ups directly under your food.

Cedarwood plank: This is a great addition to your barbecue arsenal for cooking fish. It helps infuse the fish with the flavors of the cedarwood and acts as a barrier between the fish and the heat source, which helps keep the fish moist. The cedar plank needs to be soaked in water for at least 1 hour before cooking to help it release its flavors and to prevent it from burning. If you want to pre-prep your planks, soak them in water for 1 hour, pat them lightly with paper towel to remove surface moisture, then wrap them in plastic wrap and store them in the freezer until you're ready to use them.

KEEP IN MIND

Most seafood, especially fish, is quite delicate. Avoid poking or prodding the fish too often, or it will easily break. Most seafood dishes rarely require the fish to be flipped, so as to avoid breaking it. (There are exceptions for really large pieces of fish.) Keep fish in its marinade for no more than 30 minutes. Some marinade ingredients, especially citrus, can begin to cook the fish and degrade its texture.

COMMON PROBLEMS

Overcooking. This is probably the number one problem when it comes to grilling seafood. Most fish can be finished in fewer than 15 minutes. Pay attention to the moisture level: As the fish cooks, it will start to push moisture out of the meat to the surface. For most fish, you can use a fork to test for doneness: When done, you'll just be able to start pulling the flesh away easily, but it will still maintain its firmness.

For shellfish such as lobster and shrimp, the meat will turn pink or red when it's cooked. For shellfish such as clams, mussels, and oysters, the shells will open as they cook. Once they've opened, allow them to cook a few minutes longer until the meat feels slightly firm and warm to the touch. Discard any shellfish that do not open.

ALSO TRY

Leave the skin on when cooking fish. It is a built-in insulator from the heat and can help the fish retain moisture. You can use a spatula to lift the flesh away from the skin easily after it's cooked.

SWEET CHILI SHRIMP

DIRECT HEAT COOKING
SERVES 4 ★ **PREP TIME:** 5 MINUTES ★ **COOK TIME:** 10 MINUTES
TOOLS: Vegetable grill pan (optional)

This recipe is a sweet, savory, and spicy Thai-inspired dish that is easy to make and can be done in 15 minutes. This dish features a chili-garlic sauce called sambal oelek, which is found in the international aisle of most grocery stores. It comes in a plastic jar and typically features a rooster on the label with a green lid; it should not be confused with sriracha.

FOR THE MARINADE
⅓ cup Thai sweet chili sauce
1 tablespoon sambal oelek
2 tablespoons freshly squeezed lime juice
2 tablespoons sugar
½ teaspoon kosher salt
2 pounds raw extra-jumbo (16/20) shrimp, peeled and deveined
2 tablespoons canola oil

1. In a small bowl, stir together the chili sauce, sambal oelek, lime juice, sugar, and salt.

2. Place the shrimp in a gallon-size zip-top bag and add half the marinade. Reserve the remaining marinade. Seal the bag while pressing out any air. Massage the sauce over the shrimp.

3. Preheat the grill to high heat (400°F) for direct heat cooking by lighting the heat source (or piling coals) in the spot that will be directly under the food. Put the oil on a folded paper towel and use a large pair of tongs to wipe down the grill grate with it.

4. Using the tongs, place the shrimp on the grill and discard the marinade from the bag. Grill the shrimp for 5 minutes, flip them, and grill for 4 to 5 minutes more. The shrimp are done when they start to curl and the outsides are pink.

5. Serve immediately with the reserved marinade for dipping.

EZ BBQ TIP: I like using extra-jumbo shrimp as they are really meaty and large enough not to fall through the grill grates. If you can only find smaller varieties, use a grill pan so the shrimp do not fall through the grates.

FOIL PACKET SHRIMP "BOIL"

DIRECT HEAT COOKING
SERVES 4 ★ **PREP TIME:** 15 MINUTES ★ **COOK TIME:** 15 MINUTES

This recipe modifies a New England favorite for the grill. No need to wait for giant pots of water to boil; this shrimp "boil" uses aluminum-foil packets and takes only 15 minutes to cook. The key is sealing the foil packets tightly, so they can steam the food. If you are feeling adventurous, substitute your favorite Cajun or barbecue spice for the Old Bay seasoning.

- 1 pound raw large (31/35 count) shrimp
- 1 pound baby red potatoes, halved
- 2 ears corn, husked, cut crosswise into 6 pieces
- 12 ounces andouille smoked sausage, cut into 2-inch pieces
- 4 tablespoons (½ stick) unsalted butter, melted
- 4 garlic cloves, minced
- 2 tablespoons Old Bay seasoning
- 1 teaspoon kosher salt
- ½ teaspoon freshly ground black pepper

1. Preheat the grill to medium-high heat (450°F) for direct heat cooking by lighting the heat source (or piling coals) in the spot that will be directly under the food.

2. In a large bowl, combine the shrimp, potatoes, corn, and sausage. Add the melted butter, garlic, Old Bay, salt, and pepper. Mix well to coat.

3. Place four 12-by-12-inch sheets of heavy-duty aluminum foil on a work surface and divide the ingredients among the foil sheets. Tightly seal the packets by folding up the sides over the shrimp mixture and tightly folding up the ends over the seam. (They need to be airtight, as the foil packet is used to steam the mixture.)

4. Place the foil packets on the grill and cook them for 15 minutes, or until the potatoes are fork-tender. (Carefully open one of the packets, making sure nothing spills out, to check for doneness.)

5. Serve the shrimp boil in the foil packets, so you get plenty of the spiced butter with each bite.

EZ BBQ TIP: These packets can be made ahead and kept refrigerated for up to 3 days. You can also take these on your next camping trip by freezing the packets and placing them on the grill while still frozen; they'll take 45 to 50 minutes to cook from frozen.

CAJUN BLACKENED GRILLED FISH

DIRECT HEAT COOKING
SERVES 4 ★ **PREP TIME:** 15 MINUTES + 30 MINUTES TO PREHEAT THE SKILLET ★ **COOK TIME:** 6 MINUTES
TOOLS: Baking sheet, cast-iron skillet or griddle

Blackening is a cooking technique most commonly associated with Cajun cooking. It is meant to replicate the smoky flavor of charcoal using a cast-iron skillet or griddle. The fish in this recipe is rubbed with both a spice blend and butter and is seared in a cast-iron pan until the spice blend forms a deep-brown crust. Feel free to experiment with the amount of cayenne based on your spice tolerance.

FOR THE SEASONED BUTTER

- 1 tablespoon smoked paprika
- 2 teaspoons kosher salt
- 1 teaspoon granulated garlic
- 1 teaspoon granulated onion
- 1 teaspoon cayenne pepper
- 1 teaspoon freshly ground black pepper
- ½ teaspoon dried thyme
- ½ teaspoon dried oregano
- 4 tablespoons (½ stick) unsalted butter, melted

- 4 firm white fish fillets (such as snapper, cod, or mahi-mahi; 6 to 8 ounces per fillet)
- 4 tablespoons (½ stick) unsalted butter, melted

1. In a small bowl, combine the paprika, salt, garlic, onion, cayenne, black pepper, thyme, and oregano. Add the melted butter and mix the seasoned butter well.

2. Pat each fillet dry with a paper towel and place it on a baking sheet.

3. Using your hands, evenly smear the seasoned butter all over both sides of the fillets.

4. Place a cast-iron skillet on the grill and preheat the grill to medium-high heat (450°) for direct heat cooking by lighting the heat source (or piling coals) in the spot that will be directly under the food (and the skillet, which will need to get good and hot and can take 30 minutes).

5. Once the skillet is really hot, place the fish in the skillet and cook for 2 to 3 minutes, until the bottoms of the fillets are blackened, but not burnt. Carefully flip the fillets so they do not break. Pour the melted butter over the fillets. (If you can't fit all four fillets in the skillet at the same time, cook the fish in two batches, using 2 tablespoons of melted butter for each batch.)

6. Cook the fish for 3 minutes more, or until the bottoms are blackened, but not burnt. The fish should flake easily with a fork. Transfer the fish from the skillet to a baking sheet and serve immediately.

EZ BBQ TIP: Depending on the size of your skillet and your fish, you may not be able to cook all the fillets at the same time. If this is the case, use a pair of long-handled tongs to wipe the skillet clean with a heavy-duty paper towel between batches. Scrape off any spices remaining in the skillet with a metal spatula.

GRILLED SWORDFISH WITH RED PEPPER SAUCE

DIRECT HEAT COOKING
SERVES 4 ★ PREP TIME: 15 MINUTES ★ **COOK TIME:** 25 MINUTES

This grilled swordfish features a North African harissa-style sauce and contains roasted red peppers, garlic, and Fresno chiles. A warmth and earthiness comes from the cumin and coriander. To finish this dish, I grill lemon halves, which intensifies their flavor and loosens up their juice, making them easier to squeeze.

2 tablespoons canola oil

FOR THE SAUCE

3 large red bell peppers, quartered and seeded

2 red Fresno chiles

5 tablespoons olive oil, divided

2 garlic cloves, peeled

2 teaspoons kosher salt, divided

2 teaspoons freshly ground black pepper, divided

2½ teaspoons ground cumin, divided

2½ teaspoons ground coriander, divided

4 (6-ounce) swordfish fillets

1 tablespoon plus 1 teaspoon olive oil

1 lemon, halved

1. Preheat the grill to medium-high heat (450°F) for direct heat cooking by lighting the heat source (or piling coals) in the spot that will be directly under the food. Put the canola oil on a folded paper towel and use a large pair of tongs to wipe down the grill grate with it.

2. Brush the bell peppers and Fresno chiles with 1 tablespoon of olive oil. Place the vegetables on the grill and cook for about 6 minutes per side, or until charred. Remove from the grill.

3. Carefully remove the stems and seeds from the Fresno chiles. Remove the charred skins from the bell peppers. (The skins should come off easily, but if not, place the bell peppers in a gallon-size zip-top bag or a small paper bag, seal the bag, and let the peppers steam for 10 minutes. Remove the skins.)

4. Place the vegetables in a food processor along with the garlic, 1 teaspoon of salt, 1 teaspoon of pepper, 2 teaspoons of cumin, and 2 teaspoons of coriander. Puree the vegetables while slowly adding the remaining 4 tablespoons of olive oil to the food processor.

5. Rub the fish with the olive oil and season it with the remaining 1 teaspoon of salt, the remaining 1 teaspoon of pepper, the remaining ½ teaspoon of cumin, and the remaining ½ teaspoon of coriander.

6. Place the fish on the grill and cook for 5 minutes. Place the lemon halves on the grill, cut-side down. Flip the fish and cook for 5 to 6 minutes more. The fish should flake easily while maintaining firmness. Remove the fish and lemon halves from the grill.

7. Serve the fish with the sauce spooned over it. Squeeze the lemon over the fish through a cupped hand to collect the seeds.

EZ BBQ TIP: To speed things up, you can use a store-bought harissa instead of making a sauce. Harissa is typically found in the international aisle or near the pasta sauce at your local grocery store. If you purchase harissa, start at step 4 and rub the fish with about 2 tablespoons of olive oil.

JAMAICAN JERK GRILLED HALIBUT

DIRECT HEAT COOKING
SERVES 4 ★ PREP TIME: 10 MINUTES ★ **COOK TIME:** 14 MINUTES

Spice up your next barbecue with flavors of the Caribbean. This recipe includes a homemade jerk seasoning featuring allspice, cayenne, nutmeg, and sweet paprika. I use a hearty halibut fillet that can stand up to the heat of the seasoning. Serve with the avocado to help reduce the heat factor.

FOR THE JERK RUB
3 tablespoons sweet paprika
3 tablespoons granulated garlic
1 tablespoon ground allspice
1 tablespoon kosher salt

1½ teaspoons ground nutmeg
¾ teaspoon cayenne pepper
¾ teaspoon freshly ground black pepper

4 (6-ounce) halibut fillets

½ cup pulp-free orange juice
¼ cup pineapple juice
1 tablespoon light brown sugar
2 tablespoons canola oil
2 avocados, halved, peeled, pitted, and sliced (optional)

1. In a small bowl, stir together the paprika, garlic, allspice, salt, nutmeg, cayenne, and black pepper until the rub is well combined.

2. In a gallon-size zip-top bag, combine the fillets, orange juice, pineapple juice, brown sugar, and 4 tablespoons of rub. Seal the bag while pressing out any air. Very gently massage the marinade into the fish and set aside at room temperature.

3. Preheat the grill to high heat (500°F) for direct heat cooking by lighting the heat source (or piling coals) in the spot that will be directly under the food. Put the oil on a folded paper towel and use a large pair of tongs to wipe down the grill grate with it.

4. Remove the fish from the marinade and gently pat it dry with a paper towel. Season the fish on both sides with the remaining rub.

5. Place the fish on the grill on an angle and grill for 6 minutes. Gently flip the fish with a spatula and cook for 6 to 8 minutes more, until the fish flakes easily with a fork.

6. Serve with the avocado (if using).

PARMESAN-CRUSTED GRILLED WHITEFISH

DIRECT HEAT COOKING
SERVES 4 ★ **PREP TIME:** 5 MINUTES ★ **COOK TIME:** 20 MINUTES
TOOLS: Baking sheet, zester, strainer

Growing up, I had the pleasure of fishing on Lake Michigan every summer out of Racine, Wisconsin. This dish takes me back there every time I make it. I think that whitefish is some of the best eating freshwater fish, and it is fairly firm with a large flake. If you are not able to find whitefish, use Atlantic cod or haddock.

- 1 tablespoon canola oil
- 1½ pounds whitefish fillets
- ⅔ cup panko bread crumbs
- ⅓ cup freshly grated Parmesan
- 2 tablespoons unsalted butter, at room temperature
- 2 garlic cloves, minced
- Grated zest of 1 lemon
- 1 teaspoon kosher salt
- ½ teaspoon freshly ground black pepper
- ½ teaspoon cayenne pepper
- Juice of 1 lemon

1. Preheat the grill to medium-high heat (425°F) for direct heat cooking by lighting the heat source (or piling coals) in the spot that will be directly under the food. Line a baking sheet with aluminum foil and lightly coat it with oil.

2. Place the fish on the prepared baking sheet.

3. In a small bowl, stir together the bread crumbs, Parmesan, butter, garlic, lemon zest, salt, black pepper, and cayenne. Gently press the mixture on top of the fish.

4. Place the baking sheet with the fish onto the grill and cook for about 20 minutes, until the fish flakes easily with a fork.

5. Just before serving, drizzle the lemon juice over the fish.

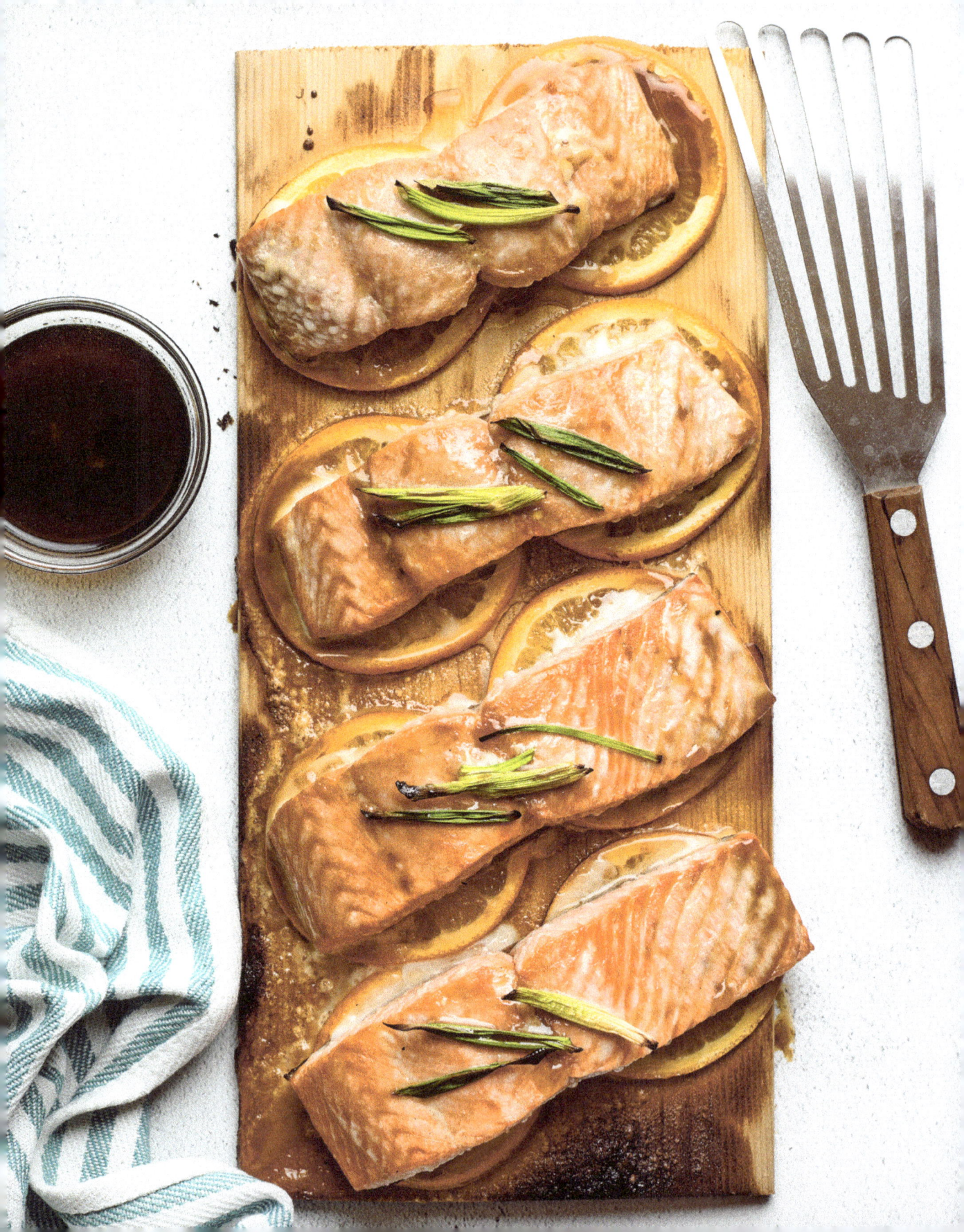

CEDAR PLANK TERIYAKI SALMON

DIRECT HEAT COOKING + STOVETOP
SERVES 4 ★ **PREP TIME:** 15 MINUTES + 1 HOUR TO SOAK THE PLANKS ★ **COOK TIME:** 20 MINUTES
TOOLS: Cedar plank, soaked in water at least 1 hour

With this recipe, I have put a twist on the classic cedar plank salmon by adding an incredibly simple homemade teriyaki sauce. It includes mirin, a sweet rice wine that is a staple in Japanese cooking. It can be found in the international aisle of your grocery store, resembles vinegar, and usually comes in a clear bottle with a red lid.

- ⅓ cup mirin (also sold as Aji-Mirin)
- 2 tablespoons low-sodium soy sauce
- 1 tablespoon sugar
- 1 navel orange
- 2 scallions, white and green parts
- 4 (6-ounce) salmon fillets

1. Preheat the grill to medium-high heat (400°F) for direct heat cooking by lighting the heat source (or piling coals) in the spot that will be directly under the food.

2. In a small saucepan on the stovetop over low heat, combine the mirin, soy sauce, and sugar and simmer for 10 minutes, stirring often, until the sauce reduces and thickens. Remove the sauce from the heat.

3. Slice the orange into eight ¼-inch rings with the peel intact. Trim off the root end of the scallions and cut them on the bias into 1-inch pieces.

4. Place the orange slices on the cedar plank two by two for the entire length of the plank. Place the salmon fillets on the orange slices. Brush half the teriyaki sauce onto the salmon and top with the scallion.

5. Place the cedar plank on the grill and close the lid. Cook for about 10 minutes until the fish flakes easily with a fork.

6. Remove the salmon from the grill and enjoy drizzled with the remaining teriyaki sauce.

EZ BBQ TIP: If you like, you can use a store-bought teriyaki sauce instead of making your own. Look for one made with minimal ingredients, especially preservatives, which impart a bitter saltiness that can overwhelm the delicate flavor of salmon.

SEAFOOD

TILAPIA PUTTANESCA

DIRECT HEAT COOKING
SERVES 4 ★ PREP TIME: 15 MINUTES ★ **COOK TIME:** 15 MINUTES

Typically, puttanesca is served as a pasta dish featuring tomatoes, olives, and capers, but I have adapted it as a light and healthy fish dish. I use tilapia, as it has a mild but slightly sweet taste that pairs well with the brininess of the capers and is contrasted by the smoky flavor of the roasted red peppers. To add a bit of savory umami, don't skip the anchovy paste.

- 4 (6- to 8-ounce) tilapia fillets
- 4 teaspoons olive oil
- ½ cup cherry tomatoes, quartered
- ½ cup pitted kalamata olives, chopped
- ½ cup roasted red peppers, chopped
- ¼ cup capers
- 2 garlic cloves, minced
- 2 teaspoons dried basil
- 1 teaspoon dried thyme
- 1 teaspoon kosher salt
- ½ teaspoon freshly ground black pepper
- ½ teaspoon anchovy paste (optional)

1. Preheat the grill to medium heat (350°F) for direct heat cooking by lighting the heat source (or piling coals) in the spot that will be directly under the food.

2. Cut out four 12-by-12-inch sheets of heavy-duty aluminum foil and place one fillet in the center of each sheet. Lightly rub the oil onto the fish.

3. In a medium bowl, stir together the tomatoes, olives, red peppers, capers, garlic, basil, thyme, salt, pepper, and anchovy paste (if using) and spoon the mixture equally over the fillets.

4. Tightly seal the foil packets by folding up the sides over the tilapia and tightly folding up the ends over the seams. (They need to be airtight, as the foil packet is used to steam the mixture.)

5. Place the foil packets on the grill and cook for about 15 minutes, until the fish is cooked through and the internal temperature reaches 150°F. The fish should flake easily with a fork. (Carefully open one of the packets, making sure nothing spills out, to check for doneness.)

6. Serve immediately.

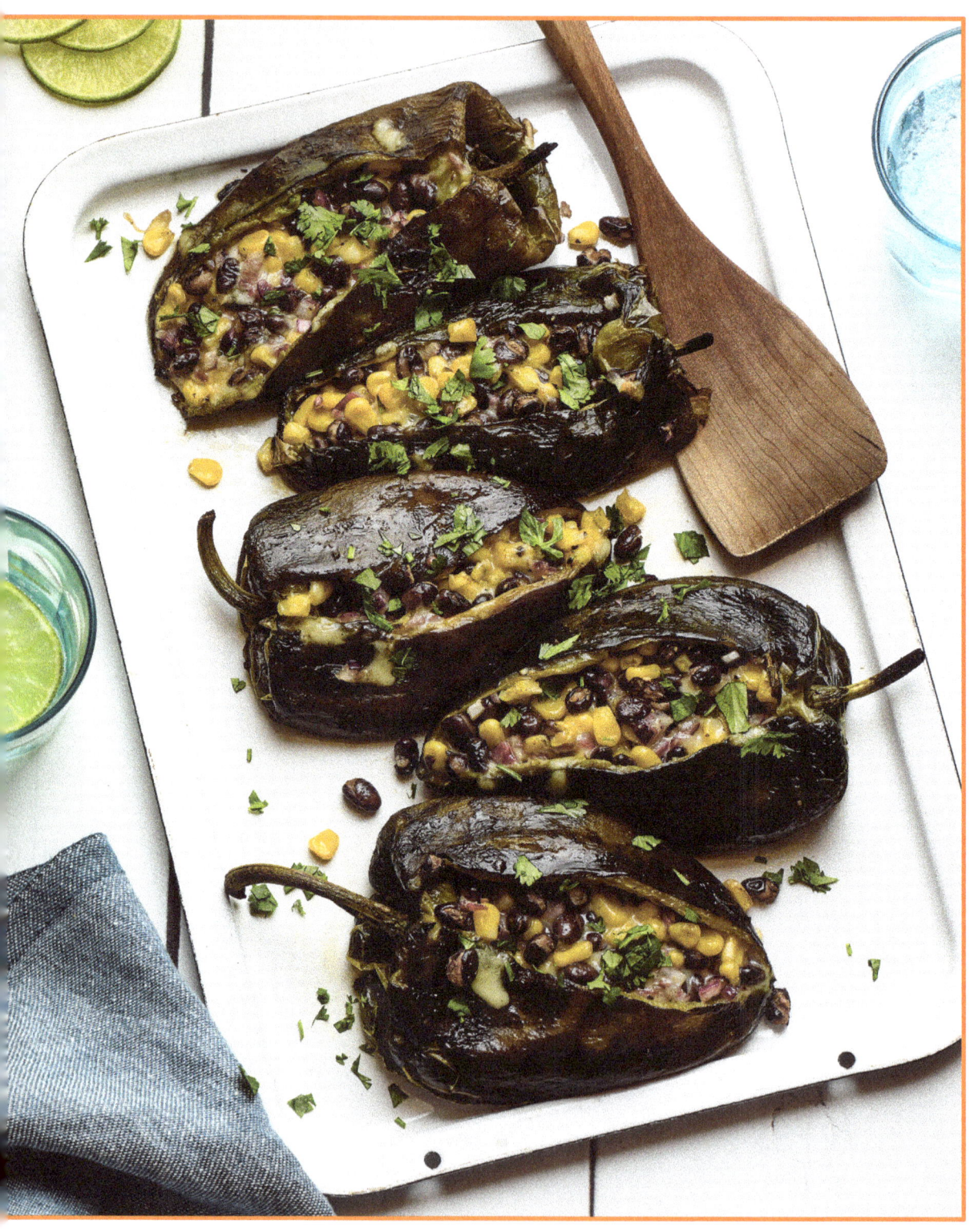

CHAPTER 6

VEGETABLES AND SIDES

GRILLED CAULIFLOWER MAC AND CHEESE **88**

HONEY-BOURBON CARROTS **90**

GREEN CHILE–CHEESE CORN BREAD **91**

GRILLED MEXICAN STREET CORN (ELOTES) **93**

GRILLED SWEET POTATOES WITH FRY SAUCE **94**

POPPA JOE'S CAMP POTATOES **96**

SMOKED FUNERAL POTATOES **97**

★ STUFFED POBLANO PEPPERS **98** ★

TWICE-COOKED PLANKED POTATOES **100**

PANCETTA-WRAPPED ASPARAGUS **102**

VEGETABLES AND SIDES CHEAT SHEET

When most people think of grilling, they think of burgers or steaks, but grilling can be a wonderful and incredibly easy way to cook vegetables, too. Most vegetables can simply be sliced, brushed with oil, and grilled over medium heat until cooked through, but there are other fun ways to prepare them as well.

BBQ COOKING STYLES

Direct heat: 350°F, medium heat 400°F to 450°F medium-high heat

Indirect heat: 350°F to 400°F, medium heat

Two-zone indirect heat: 350°F, medium heat, for casseroles

DONENESS CUES

Typically, a vegetable is fully cooked when it can be pierced with a fork easily but does not split or break at the spot it's been poked.

★ When grilling corn, prick a kernel with the tip of a sharp knife; it should squirt out some of its juice.

★ When cooking mushrooms, look for a slightly golden-brown color but make sure they are still pliable and moist.

USEFUL TOOLS

Vegetable grill pan: A grilling pan—which looks like a perforated baking sheet, with holes to allow oils and liquids to drain away and heat to pass through—can be a real lifesaver for grilled vegetables. Many good vegetables have been lost between the grates when they're flipped. Place the pan on the grill about 5 minutes before putting your vegetables on, to get the pan up to temperature, which keeps the vegetable from sticking to it.

Mandoline slicer: The key to cooking vegetables evenly is to keep their size consistent. Pieces that vary greatly in size take different times to cook. For vegetables that can be sliced, a mandoline is invaluable because it creates extremely consistent slices. Set the slicer to cut pieces about ¼ inch thick. Depending on the vegetable, you can get creative and cut them lengthwise, so you get longer strips instead of rounds.

KEEP IN MIND

Leave the grill cover open. If you close it, the vegetable will bake and get mushy. If you're using a charcoal grill, closing the lid can also cause the vegetables to get overly smoky, ruining their delicate flavor.

Don't touch them! Most vegetables need to be cooked on two sides, but don't touch them once you put them on the grill. Allow the vegetables to get grill marks as their natural sugars to caramelize. Constantly touching the vegetables before they char will cause them to stick to the grate and mess up those beautiful grill marks. Once they're fully cooked on one side, they'll be easier to flip to cook the second side.

COMMON PROBLEMS

Dry vegetables: Keep veggies from drying out by soaking them in water before grilling. Thoroughly dry them with a paper towel after they've been soaked, so they still char.
Uneven cooking: To prevent uneven cooking, chop all your vegetables to the same size. (But don't make them too small or they will fall through the grill grate.)

ALSO TRY

Fire Roasting: A quick way to transform the flavor of your vegetables completely is to fire roast them. This method is best for vegetables with skin, such as peppers, tomatoes, and eggplants. Make sure the grill is at its highest setting and grill the vegetables over direct heat until they start to char. If you have a charcoal grill, roast the vegetables directly on the embers.

GRILLED CAULIFLOWER MAC AND CHEESE

DIRECT HEAT COOKING + STOVETOP
SERVES 4 ★ **PREP TIME:** 15 MINUTES ★ **COOK TIME:** 25 MINUTES
TOOL: Vegetable grill pan

This twist on traditional mac and cheese, which is great as either a side or main course, uses grilled cauliflower instead of elbow macaroni. The cauliflower creates a completely different texture, and the char from the grill brings the flavor to a new level. I suggest buying a whole cheese block and grating it yourself, as pre-shredded cheese contains ingredients to keep it from clumping, which can also prevent it from melting well.

- 2 tablespoons canola oil
- 2 large heads cauliflower (about 4 pounds)
- 1 tablespoon olive oil
- 1 teaspoon kosher salt
- ½ teaspoon granulated garlic
- 4 tablespoons (½ stick) cold unsalted butter
- ½ cup all-purpose flour
- 2 cups whole milk
- 2 teaspoons mustard powder (preferably Colman's brand)
- 1 teaspoon freshly ground black pepper
- 1 teaspoon hot sauce (such as Texas Pete's)
- 3 cups shredded sharp cheddar cheese

1. Preheat the grill to medium heat (350°F) for direct heat cooking by lighting the heat source (or piling coals) in the spot that will be directly under the food. Put the oil on a folded paper towel and use a large pair of tongs to wipe down the grill grate with it.

2. Remove the outer leaves from each cauliflower head, remove the stem from the bottom of the cauliflower, and stand it upright on the cutting board. Using a large, sharp knife, cut each cauliflower head into 4 large pieces, or steaks. Brush both sides of the cauliflower steaks with the olive oil and season with the salt and garlic.

3. Place the cauliflower steaks on the grill and close the lid. Cook for 5 to 6 minutes, until the bottom of the steaks begins to char, then carefully flip the steaks and cook for 5 minutes more, until tender.

4. Remove the cauliflower from the grill and cut the steaks into florets.

5. In a large saucepan on the stovetop over medium heat, melt the butter. Whisk in the flour and cook for 3 to 4 minutes until golden brown, whisking occasionally. While whisking, slowly pour in the milk and whisk until fully combined. Whisk in the mustard powder, pepper, and hot sauce. Simmer the mixture for about 5 minutes, until it begins to thicken.

6. Turn off the heat and stir in the cheese until it is completely melted. Stir in the cauliflower and gently toss until fully coated in the cheese sauce.

EZ BBQ TIP: If your cauliflower is a bit crumbly and you're concerned it will fall apart on the grill, use a vegetable grill pan. Place the pan on the grill during the preheating stage, in step 1, to ensure it is hot, then cook the cauliflower steaks on it.

HONEY-BOURBON CARROTS

TWO-ZONE DIRECT AND INDIRECT HEAT COOKING + STOVETOP
SERVES 6 ★ **PREP TIME:** 10 MINUTES ★ **COOK TIME:** 35 MINUTES
TOOLS: Hickory or apple wood chips (optional)

This dish is one of my favorite ways to jazz up what I feel is a pretty boring vegetable. The charred carrots combine perfectly with the sweetness of the honey and the oaky taste of the bourbon. The optional use of hickory or apple wood will further enhance the grilled flavor of these carrots. Finish them with a sprinkle of fresh thyme leaves to round off the dish.

FOR THE GLAZE
3 tablespoons cold unsalted butter
3 tablespoons honey
3 tablespoons bourbon

2 pounds whole carrots (preferably with tops)
1 teaspoon kosher salt
1 teaspoon freshly ground black pepper

1 teaspoon fresh thyme leaves

1. Preheat the grill to medium heat (350°F) for two-zone indirect heat cooking by lighting the heat source (or piling coals) on one side of the grill. Add a handful of hickory or apple wood chips to the grill (if using).

2. In a small saucepan on the stovetop over medium-low heat, melt the butter. Add the honey and bourbon and stir until they are fully incorporated. Simmer the glaze for 5 minutes, until it thickens. Remove it from the heat.

3. If your carrots have tops, cut them down to about 1 inch. If your carrots are really large, you may need to halve them lengthwise, so they cook evenly.

4. Brush the carrots with the glaze, season them with the salt and pepper, place them over direct heat on the grill, and close the lid. Cook the carrots for about 10 minutes, turning them with a pair of long-handled tongs and brushing them with more glaze every 2 minutes, until they are slightly charred all over.

5. Transfer the carrots to the indirect side of the grill, brush them with more glaze, and close the lid. Cook the carrots for 15 to 17 minutes, until they are fork-tender. Remove the carrots from the grill.

6. Drizzle the carrots with the remaining glaze and sprinkle with the thyme leaves before serving.

GREEN CHILE-CHEESE CORN BREAD

INDIRECT HEAT COOKING
SERVES 5 ★ **PREP TIME:** 15 MINUTES ★ **COOK TIME:** 35 MINUTES
TOOLS: 9-by-9-inch baking dish

My wife, Vida, was born and raised in Arizona, and corn bread was a staple in her household. After we were married, she adapted her mother's recipe for corn bread for the grill and added green chiles and shredded cheese. Vida has kept this recipe pretty close and hasn't shared it much outside the family, but she let me take a sneak peek at it, and now I am sharing it with you. I love drizzlingly a bit of honey on my slice and eating it hot, right off the grill.

Nonstick cooking spray
1 cup all-purpose flour
1 cup yellow cornmeal
¼ cup sugar
2½ teaspoons baking powder
½ teaspoon kosher salt
1 cup whole milk
1 (14.75-ounce) can cream-style corn
4 tablespoons (½ stick) unsalted butter, melted
2 large eggs, beaten
1 (4-ounce) can fire-roasted diced green chiles
½ cup shredded Mexican-style cheese blend

1. Preheat the grill to medium heat (400°F) for indirect cooking.
2. Lightly coat a 9-by-9-inch baking dish with cooking spray.
3. In a medium bowl, whisk the flour, cornmeal, sugar, baking powder, and salt well.
4. In another medium bowl, stir together the milk, corn, melted butter, eggs, green chiles, and cheese until well combined. Pour the wet ingredients into the dry ingredients and gently stir to combine. There should be no signs of flour in the mixture when finished (don't overwork the batter). Transfer the batter to the prepared baking dish and place it on the indirect side of the grill.
5. Cook for 15 minutes. Rotate the pan 180 degrees and cook for 15 to 20 minutes more, until a butter knife inserted into the center of the corn bread comes out clean.
6. Slice the corn bread into squares and serve warm.

VARIATION TIP: For a twist, instead of the yellow cornmeal, use blue cornmeal. It has a more flavorful corn taste, is slightly sweeter, and can be a bit crumblier.

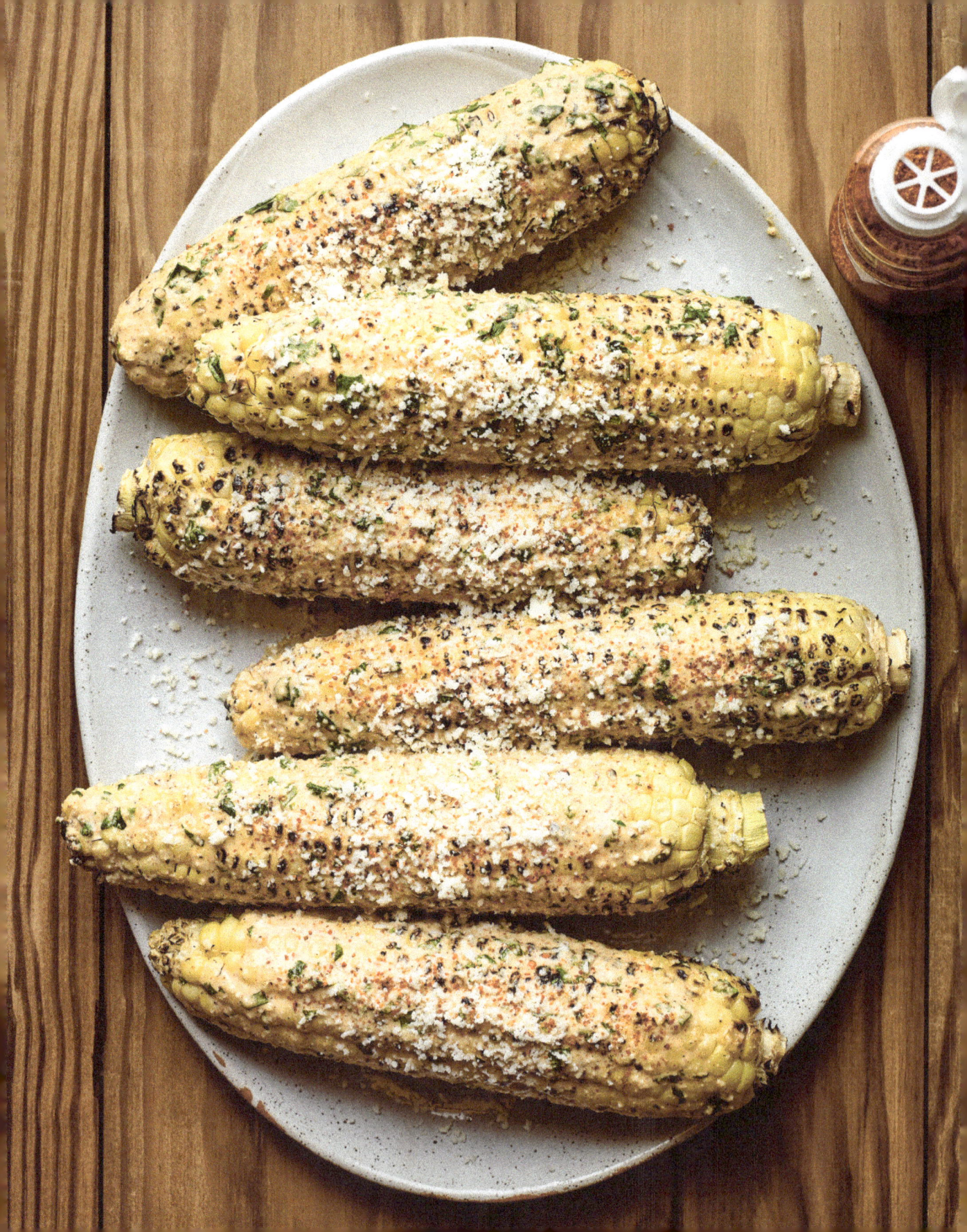

GRILLED MEXICAN STREET CORN (ELOTES)

DIRECT HEAT COOKING
SERVES 4 ★ **PREP TIME:** 10 MINUTES ★ **COOK TIME:** 12 MINUTES

Elotes, also known as Mexican street corn, is a dish of grilled corn on the cob slathered in mayonnaise and flavored with cilantro, chili powder, lime juice, and salty cotija cheese. This dish is popular all over Mexico and throughout the western United States. The cotija cheese can be found in most supermarkets and is similar in taste to Parmesan. I suggest finding it whole and grating it yourself to get the freshest flavor.

- 3 tablespoons canola oil, divided
- 6 ears sweet corn, husked
- 1 teaspoon kosher salt
- ¾ cup grated cotija cheese, divided
- ½ cup chopped fresh cilantro leaves
- ¼ cup mayonnaise
- 1 tablespoon freshly squeezed lime juice
- 1 teaspoon granulated garlic
- ½ teaspoon freshly ground black pepper
- ½ teaspoon chili powder
- Tajín seasoning, for garnish (optional)

1. Preheat the grill to medium-high heat (450°F) for direct heat cooking by lighting the heat source (or piling coals) in the spot that will be directly under the food. Put 2 tablespoons of oil on a folded paper towel and use a large pair of tongs to wipe down the grill grate with it.

2. Brush the corn with the remaining 1 tablespoon of oil and season it with salt. Put the corn on the grill and cook it for 10 to 12 minutes, flipping every 2 to 3 minutes to char each side. Test for doneness by pricking a kernel with the tip of a sharp knife and watch for it to squirt out its juice.

3. In a medium bowl large enough to fit an ear of corn, stir together ½ cup of cotija cheese, the cilantro, mayonnaise, lime juice, garlic, pepper, and chili powder.

4. Working with one ear at a time, place the corn in the bowl and roll it around until it is completely covered in the cheese mixture. Top the seasoned corn with the remaining cotija cheese and garnish with Tajín (if using).

VARIATION TIP: Kick this dish up with some smoky heat by adding 2 tablespoons of adobo sauce (from a can of chipotles in adobo sauce) to the mayonnaise mixture in step 3.

GRILLED SWEET POTATOES WITH FRY SAUCE

DIRECT HEAT COOKING + MICROWAVE
SERVES 4 ★ PREP TIME: 15 MINUTES ★ **COOK TIME:** 18 MINUTES
TOOLS: Microwave

As someone who has lived in the western states for the majority of my adult life, I have driven through Utah numerous times. Every time, I find myself seeking out burger joints that serve "fry sauce." This wonderful condiment is made of one part ketchup and two parts mayonnaise and seasoned with a few other ingredients that amp up the flavor. I have found that this sauce goes really well with slightly charred grilled sweet potatoes—the combination of sweetness, char, and tang is perfectly balanced.

4 large sweet potatoes

FOR THE FRY SAUCE
1 cup mayonnaise
½ cup ketchup
1½ tablespoons dill pickle juice

1½ teaspoons Worcestershire sauce
1 teaspoon sweet paprika
½ teaspoon cayenne pepper

3 tablespoons olive oil
1 teaspoon kosher salt
1 teaspoon freshly ground black pepper
1 teaspoon dried rosemary

1. Clean the sweet potatoes and then pierce them with a fork. Place the sweet potatoes on a microwave-safe plate and microwave on high power, uncovered, for 6 to 8 minutes, turning once. They are ready when a fork inserted into the potato still gives some resistance.

2. In a medium bowl, whisk the mayonnaise, ketchup, pickle juice, Worcestershire sauce, paprika, and cayenne to combine thoroughly. Cover the bowl and refrigerate the sauce to allow the flavors to blend.

3. Preheat the grill to medium-high heat (450°F) for direct heat cooking by lighting the heat source (or piling coals) in the spot that will be directly under the food.

4. Carefully—they will be hot—slice the sweet potatoes into ½-inch-thick rounds. Brush both sides of the slices with oil and season with the salt, black pepper, and rosemary.

5. Place the potatoes on the grill. Cook for 4 to 5 minutes, or until you see grill marks. Flip the slices and cook for 4 to 5 minutes more. The sweet potatoes are done when both sides have grill marks and the potatoes are pierced easily with a fork.

6. Serve with the fry sauce for dipping.

VARIATION TIP: I am a huge fan of sambal oelek, a chili-garlic sauce from Southeast Asia, and I love adding 1 tablespoon to my fry sauce in step 2 with the other ingredients.

POPPA JOE'S CAMP POTATOES

DIRECT HEAT COOKING
SERVES 4 ★ PREP TIME: 10 MINUTES ★ **COOK TIME:** 30 MINUTES

Every summer, my dad and I would go camping on St. Martin Island in Lake Michigan, near Door County, Wisconsin. In the evenings, we would grill up the day's catch of salmon on the beach with a side of his camp potatoes. According to my dad, I had an unrefined palette as a kid and didn't like any spices other than salt and pepper. Thankfully, I have grown up a bit since then, and over the years, I have modified this childhood favorite to include an assortment of herbs.

- **2 large russet potatoes, skin on, cut into 1-inch cubes**
- **1 medium white onion, chopped**
- **2 tablespoons unsalted butter, melted**
- **2 tablespoons canola oil**
- **2 teaspoons dried rosemary**
- **2 teaspoons dried basil**
- **2 teaspoons dried thyme**
- **2 teaspoons kosher salt**
- **1 teaspoon freshly ground black pepper**
- **4 garlic cloves, peeled**

1. Preheat the grill to medium-high heat (400°F) for direct heat cooking by lighting the heat source (or piling coals) in the spot that will be directly under the food.

2. In a large bowl, combine the potatoes, onion, melted butter, oil, rosemary, basil, thyme, salt, and pepper.

3. Tear two 12-by-18-inches sheets of heavy-duty aluminum foil and place them on your work surface. Divide the potato mixture evenly between the sheets and add 2 garlic cloves to each pile. Fold up the sides of the foil, tightly sealing them to create foil packets.

4. Lay the foil packets on the grill with the seal facing up. Cook for 25 to 30 minutes, until the potatoes are tender (carefully open the packets to test for doneness). The potatoes should be golden brown and pierce easily with a fork.

VARIATION TIP: There are so many possibilities with this dish. Some of my favorite variations include adding ¼ cup of diced roasted red pepper to the mixture, or add 2 teaspoons of finely diced jalapeño for a spicy kick. Add 2 tablespoons of regular or spicy ranch dressing for a tangy, creamier version. If you do not have russets, Yukon Gold or red potatoes also work.

SMOKED FUNERAL POTATOES

DIRECT HEAT COOKING
SERVES 4 ★ PREP TIME: 10 MINUTES ★ **COOK TIME:** 1 HOUR 30 MINUTES
TOOLS: Apple or hickory wood chips (optional), 12-inch cast-iron skillet

Funeral potatoes are a cheesy casserole dish that originated in the western United States as a comfort food served at gatherings held after funerals. The dish's popularity has grown, and now it's a regular component of potlucks and family gatherings. The ingredients are fairly dense and take at least a good hour to cook through fully.

Nonstick cooking spray
1 (32-ounce) package frozen hash browns
2 cups grated sharp cheddar cheese
1½ cups sour cream
1 (10.5-ounce) can cream of chicken soup
2 tablespoons grated Parmesan cheese
2 garlic cloves, minced
1 teaspoon smoked paprika
½ teaspoon freshly ground black pepper
1½ cups roughly-crushed cornflakes cereal
4 tablespoons (½ stick) unsalted butter, melted

1. Preheat the grill to medium heat (350°F) for direct heat cooking by lighting the heat source (or piling coals) in the spot that will be directly under the food. Add a handful of apple or hickory wood chips to the grill (if using). Lightly coat a 12-inch cast-iron skillet with cooking spray.

2. In large bowl, stir together the hash browns, cheddar, sour cream, soup, Parmesan, garlic, paprika, and pepper. Transfer the mixture to the prepared skillet.

3. In a small bowl, stir together the cornflakes and melted butter. Sprinkle this mixture over the potato mixture.

4. Place the skillet on the grill, close the lid, and cook for 1 to 1½ hours, or until the potatoes are tender. If the cornflakes start to brown too much before the potatoes are cooked through, cover the pan with aluminum foil until the potatoes finish cooking.

EZ BBQ TIP: If you do not want to keep an eye on the grill the whole 1½ hours while this dish cooks, cook it for 20 minutes on the grill to absorb some of the smoke flavor and then finish it in a 350°F oven for another hour, or until the potatoes are tender.

STUFFED POBLANO PEPPERS

DIRECT HEAT COOKING + STOVETOP
SERVES 6 ★ PREP TIME: 10 MINUTES ★ **COOK TIME:** 25 MINUTES

Poblano peppers are a mild variety of chile pepper popular in Mexico. They are little larger than a bell pepper, and on the spice scale, they are between a bell pepper and an Anaheim chile. Grilling the poblanos makes them slightly sweet and adds a bit of smoky flavor from the charring. If you are concerned about the spiciness of this dish, use bell peppers instead.

- 2 tablespoons canola oil
- 6 medium poblano peppers
- 2 tablespoons cold unsalted butter
- ½ medium red onion, finely chopped
- 1 (15-ounce) can black beans, drained and rinsed
- 2 cups frozen corn kernels
- ¼ cup fresh cilantro, chopped
- 2 garlic cloves, minced
- 1½ teaspoons kosher salt
- 1 teaspoon ground cumin
- ¼ teaspoon freshly ground black pepper
- 2 cups shredded Monterey Jack cheese
- Nonstick cooking spray

1. Preheat the grill to medium-high heat (400°F) for direct heat cooking by lighting the heat source (or piling coals) in the spot that will be directly under the food. Put the oil on a folded paper towel and use a large pair of tongs to wipe down the grill grate with it.

2. Place the poblano peppers on the grill and close the lid. Cook for about 10 minutes, turning the peppers once, until the skins are charred. Transfer the peppers to a gallon-size zip-top bag or a small paper bag. Seal the bag and let the peppers steam in the bag for 10 minutes.

3. Meanwhile, in a large skillet on the stovetop over medium-high heat, melt the butter. Add the onion and cook for about 5 minutes until translucent. Stir in the black beans and corn. Add the cilantro, garlic, salt, cumin, and pepper and stir until well-combined. Cook until the mixture begins to bubble, remove the skillet from the heat, and stir in the cheese.

4. Remove the poblanos from the bag. Gently peel off and discard the skins, keeping the stems attached to the peppers. Make a lengthwise slit down the side of each pepper, being careful not to cut through to the other side. Use a teaspoon to gently remove the peppers' seeds and membranes.

5. Lightly coat a baking sheet with cooking spray and place the poblanos on it. Spoon the corn and bean mixture evenly into the poblanos. Pull the sides of the peppers around the filling to close them.

6. Place the baking sheet on the grill, close the lid, and cook the peppers for 5 minutes, until the cheese is melted and bubbling. Remove the peppers from the grill and serve immediately.

TWICE-COOKED PLANKED POTATOES

STOVETOP + INDIRECT HEAT COOKING
SERVES 4 ★ **PREP TIME:** 5 MINUTES ★ **COOK TIME:** 45 MINUTES
TOOLS: Cedar plank (soaked in water for at least 1 hour), apple or hickory wood chips (optional), potato masher or electric hand mixer

I am a huge fan of potatoes, and this recipe joins the flavors of two favorites: loaded baked potato and twice-baked potato. Using a cedar plank to cook the potatoes—and adding some wood chips, if you like—gives the dish a nice smoky flavor.

- 4 medium russet potatoes, skin on, cut into 1-inch cubes
- 2 teaspoons kosher salt, divided
- 6 tablespoons (¾ stick) unsalted butter, at room temperature
- 4 ounces cream cheese, at room temperature, cut into slices
- 1 tablespoon dried rosemary
- 1 scallion, white and green parts, thinly sliced
- 1 teaspoon freshly ground black pepper
- ⅓ cup whole milk
- ⅓ cup shredded sharp cheddar cheese
- 3 bacon slices, cooked and chopped (optional)

1. In a medium saucepan on the stovetop over high heat, combine the potatoes with enough cold water to cover and 1 teaspoon of salt. Bring to a boil, then reduce the heat to medium and cook the potatoes for 15 to 20 minutes, until they are fork-tender. Drain the potatoes and return them to the pan. Place the pot over low heat and cook the potatoes for about 2 minutes, stirring, to remove any remaining moisture.

2. With the pan still over low heat, mash the potatoes. Stir in the butter, cream cheese, rosemary, scallion, remaining 1 teaspoon of salt, and pepper until fully incorporated. Add the milk and mix until it is fully absorbed and the potatoes are creamy.

3. Preheat the grill to medium heat (350°F) for indirect heat cooking by lighting only the heat source (or piling coals) across from where you will place the food. Add a handful of apple or hickory wood to your grill (if using).

4. Mound the potatoes on the cedar plank and top them with the cheese.

5. Place the cedar plank on the indirect heat side of the grill, close the lid, and cook the potatoes for 20 minutes. When finished, the potatoes should have some brown edges and the cheese should be fully melted. Top the potatoes with the bacon (if using) and serve.

> **EZ BBQ TIP:** To save some time, cook the potatoes in the microwave, in a covered glass bowl, for 7 to 9 minutes on high power, or until they can be pierced easily with a fork. Pick up the recipe at step 2.

PANCETTA-WRAPPED ASPARAGUS

DIRECT HEAT COOKING
SERVES 4 ★ **PREP TIME:** 10 MINUTES ★ **COOK TIME:** 6 MINUTES
TOOLS: Vegetable grill pan (optional)

This recipe is a spin on the classic dish of asparagus with prosciutto. It uses pancetta, a salt-cured pork belly that is similar to bacon but is rolled and placed in a casing before it's cured. Unlike prosciutto, it is raw and needs to be cooked before it's eaten, but in the end it cooks up crispier due to its higher fat content. The pancetta's salty, porky flavor provides a nice balance to the earthy flavor of the asparagus. This incredibly easy side dish is a crowd-pleaser.

- 2 tablespoons canola oil
- 12 medium asparagus spears
- 1 tablespoon olive oil
- ½ teaspoon freshly ground black pepper
- 12 pancetta slices

1. Preheat the grill to medium-high heat (400°F) for direct heat cooking by lighting the heat source (or piling coals) in the spot that will be directly under the food. Put the canola oil on a folded paper towel and use a large pair of tongs to wipe down the grill grate with it.

2. Trim off the woody ends of the asparagus (about an inch) and place the spears on a plate. Drizzle the asparagus with the olive oil and toss until it is fully coated. Season the asparagus with the pepper. Wrap the middle of each spear with 1 pancetta slice.

3. Place the asparagus on the grill across the grates (so they do not fall in) or use a vegetable grill pan. Cook for about 6 minutes, uncovered, turning every minute, until the pancetta is fully cooked and the asparagus is tender.

4. Remove from the grill and serve immediately.

VARIATION TIP: If you are looking to impress folks, substitute purple asparagus for the traditional green asparagus. It's typically only found in springtime, and you may have to hunt around at your higher-end grocery store to find it. It is often more tender and less fibrous than its green counterpart.

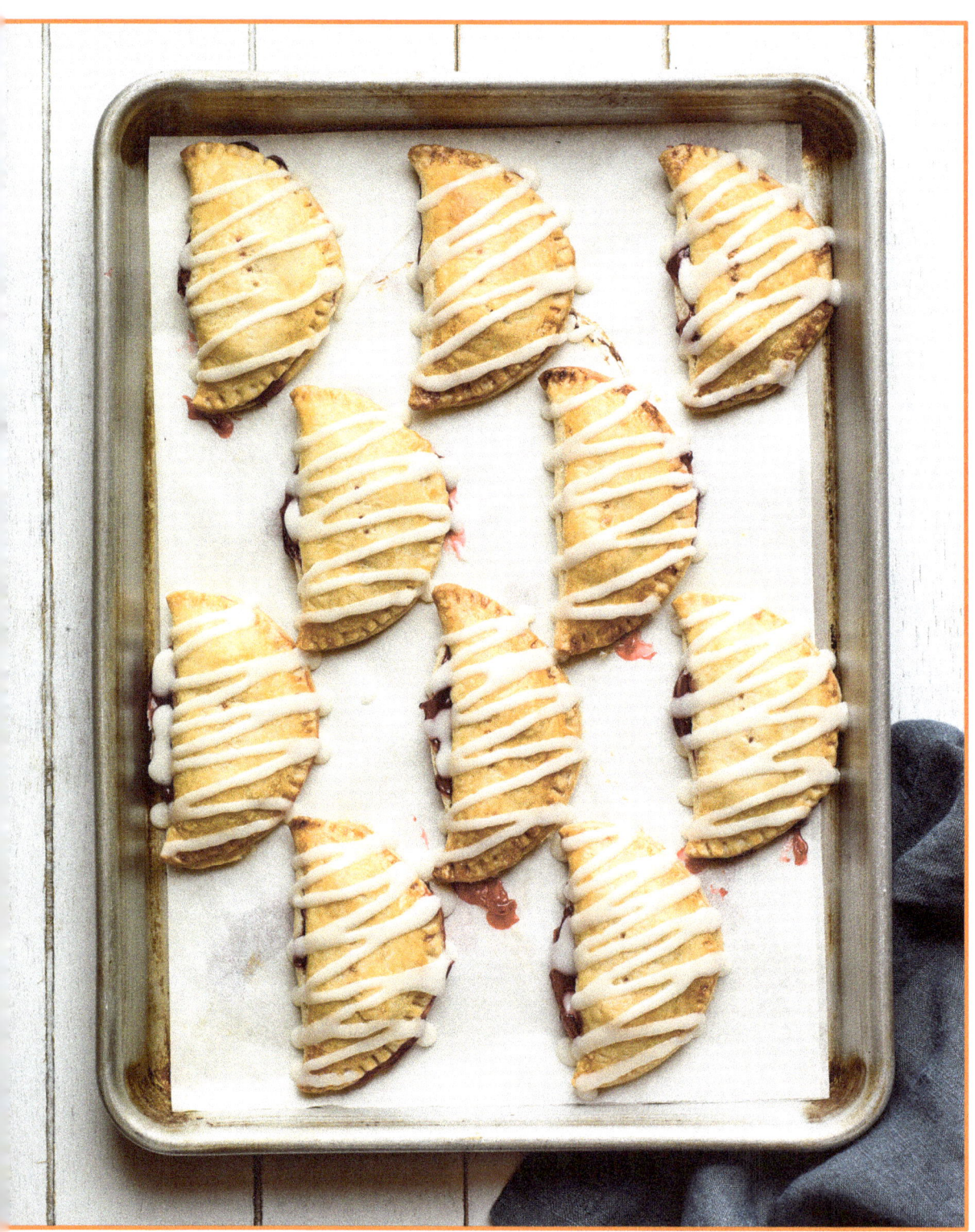

CHAPTER 7

DESSERTS

BLUEBERRY AND PEACH GALETTE **108**

GRILLED S'MORES DIP **109**

PINEAPPLE UPSIDE-DOWN CAKE **110**

SMOKY BAKED APPLES **112**

TRIPLE-BERRY CRISP **113**

★ GRILLED CHERRY HAND PIES **114** ★

DESSERTS CHEAT SHEET

Making desserts on the grill can be quite easy with a little bit of practice for temperature control. Your outdoor grill should be an extension of your kitchen, and using it for all the elements of your meal allows you to take advantage of the fact that the grill is already preheated, so you can transition quickly to dessert without having to move inside to finish cooking.

BBQ COOKING STYLES

Direct heat:
350°F to 400°F, medium heat
425°F, medium-high heat

Indirect heat:
350°F, medium heat

DONENESS CUES

★ Cooked fruit should be soft and bubbling.

★ Cake batter is cooked through when a tester inserted into the middle comes out clean.

★ Pastry dough is done when golden brown and flaky.

USEFUL TOOLS

Cast-iron skillet: A cast-iron skillet is an invaluable tool when cooking desserts on the grill. The thick cast iron allows desserts to cook slowly and adapts to temperature fluctuations better than thin aluminum or stainless-steel cookware. The ability to hold heat evenly also provides a consistent cook.

Temperature probe: When baking on a grill, it is important to have really good temperature control. Using a probe (ideally with remote monitoring capability) will help you keep an eye on the temperature while still being able to do other things.

KEEP IN MIND

Not too hot: As fruit contains sugar, it can easily burn if cooked at higher temperatures. Before cooking, take the time to make sure that the temperature has stabilized to your desired level.

Avoid extra moisture. Fruit also has a lot of moisture, which can lead to soggy pastries or filling. Unless the recipe calls for a different approach, be sure to thaw frozen fruit fully and pat it dry with a paper towel to remove unwanted moisture.

COMMON PROBLEMS

Burnt desserts: In some grills, the heat source can be too close to the grill grate, which can cause desserts to burn. If this is the case with your grill, cook the recipe using an indirect heat method, so the heat source is not directly under the food. If your grill is large enough, place the dessert in the center of the grill with only the side burners lit. The same setup can be done on a charcoal grill—push the charcoal to the sides of the grill and place the dessert in the center.

ALSO TRY

Grilled Fruit: For a quick dessert, grill fruits such as peaches, pineapple, plums, nectarines, and watermelon directly on the grill. Using a direct heat cooking setup at medium-high heat (450°F), place the fruit directly on the grill and cook it for 3 to 5 minutes, then flip it over and cook for 3 to 5 minutes more. The fruit should be warmed through and have grill marks when done.

BLUEBERRY AND PEACH GALETTE

DIRECT HEAT COOKING + MICROWAVE

SERVES 8 ★ **PREP TIME:** 15 MINUTES + 20 MINUTES TO REST ★ **COOK TIME:** 30 MINUTES
TOOLS: Baking sheet, parchment paper, apple wood chips (optional), microwave, cooling rack

This recipe is inspired by late-summer peaches and blueberries. The fruit is wrapped in a free-form crust and grilled until the fruit is soft, the crust is golden brown, and everything is delicious.

- 1 (14-ounce) package refrigerated (not frozen in the tin) piecrust (contains 2 piecrusts)
- 5 fresh peaches, cut into ½-inch slices
- 1 cup fresh blueberries
- ¼ cup packed light brown sugar
- 2 tablespoons all-purpose flour
- ¼ teaspoon ground cinnamon
- ⅛ teaspoon ground nutmeg
- Pinch kosher salt
- 2 tablespoons unsalted butter, melted
- 3 tablespoons apricot preserves

1. Line a baking sheet with parchment paper. Remove the piecrusts from the refrigerator and let them come to room temperature. Meanwhile, in a medium bowl, gently mix the peaches, blueberries, brown sugar, flour, cinnamon, nutmeg, and salt. Add the melted butter and mix again.

2. Preheat the grill to medium heat (400°F) for direct heat cooking by lighting the heat source (or piling coals) in the spot that will be directly under the food. Add a handful of apple wood chips to the grill (if using).

3. Transfer one piecrust to one side of the prepared baking sheet. Place half of the peach mixture into the center of the crust and spread it evenly, leaving a 1½-inch border all the way around. Fold the border of the crust over, working your way around the edge and creating a pleat about every 3 inches. Repeat the process with the remaining piecrust and filling.

4. In a small microwave-safe bowl, warm the apricot preserves in the microwave for 15 to 20 seconds until soft. Brush the preserves onto the galette crusts.

5. Place the baking sheet on the grill and cook the galettes for 15 minutes. Rotate the pan 180 degrees and grill for 15 minutes more. The crusts should be lightly browned. Carefully transfer the galettes to a cooling rack, and let them rest for 20 minutes or longer.

GRILLED S'MORES DIP

INDIRECT HEAT COOKING
SERVES 4 ★ **PREP TIME:** 5 MINUTES ★ **COOK TIME:** 20 MINUTES
TOOLS: Cast-iron skillet

This recipe transforms a summertime classic into a less-messy dessert that lets you skip the sticks and serve all your guests at once. In this method, chocolate chips are topped with marshmallows and then grilled until golden brown, forming a thick dip you can scoop up with a graham cracker "spoon." Nothing screams summertime like s'mores.

- 1 tablespoon canola oil
- 1 (23-ounce) bag milk chocolate chips
- 1½ cups mini marshmallows
- 9 graham crackers, each broken into 4 pieces (36 crackers total)

1. Preheat the grill to medium heat (350°) for indirect heat cooking by lighting only the heat source (or piling coals) across from where you will place the food.

2. Put the oil on a folded paper towel and coat the inside of a cast-iron skillet with it. Line the bottom of the skillet with the chocolate chips, spreading them evenly. Top the chocolate with the marshmallows.

3. Place the skillet on the indirect side of the grill and cook for 15 to 20 minutes, or until the chocolate has melted and the marshmallows are lightly toasted.

4. Remove the skillet from the grill and serve the dip right away with the graham crackers to scoop up the dip.

VARIATION TIP: Experiment with different types of chocolate chips, such as semi-sweet, white, and dark. If the dessert feels too sweet, add 1 cup of fresh blueberries between the chocolate and marshmallow topping.

PINEAPPLE UPSIDE-DOWN CAKE

DIRECT HEAT COOKING

SERVES 12 ★ **PREP TIME:** 10 MINUTES ★ **COOK TIME:** 40 MINUTES + 1 HOUR TO COOL
TOOLS: 9-by-13-inch nonstick baking dish, stand mixer, strainer

This adaptation of a traditional upside-down cake is the ideal grilled dessert for pineapple lovers. My recipe includes crushed pineapple on top of the cake and pineapple juice in the batter, so you get fruit in each bite. The finished cake has a caramelized top, from the sugar and pineapple cooking right in the pan, and bright-red maraschino cherries peeking through.

- 1 (20-ounce) can crushed pineapple in 100% pineapple juice
- 2¼ cups all-purpose flour
- 1½ cups granulated sugar
- 3½ teaspoons baking powder
- 1 teaspoon salt
- 8 tablespoons (1 stick) unsalted butter, at room temperature, plus 4 tablespoons (½ stick), melted
- 1¼ cups whole milk
- 2 tablespoons vegetable oil
- 1 tablespoon vanilla extract
- 3 large eggs
- 1 cup packed light brown sugar
- 12 maraschino cherries

1. Preheat the grill to medium heat (350°F) for direct heat cooking by lighting the heat source (or piling coals) in the spot that will be directly under the food.

2. Pour the crushed pineapple into a strainer set over a bowl and push the pineapple down using the back of a spoon to remove most of the liquid. Reserve the pineapple juice.

3. In a medium bowl, whisk the flour, granulated sugar, baking powder, and salt.

4. Place 8 tablespoons (1 stick) of room-temperature butter into the bowl of a stand mixer fitted with the paddle attachment and beat on medium speed for 1 to 2 minutes, until creamy. Add the dry ingredients to the butter and beat for about 30 seconds until combined. Pour in the milk (replacing as much of the milk as possible with the reserved pineapple juice), oil, vanilla, and eggs. Beat on medium speed for 1 to 2 minutes, until fully incorporated.

5. Pour the tablespoons of melted butter into a 9-by-13-inch baking dish and fully coat the surface. Pour in the brown sugar and spread it evenly over the bottom of the dish. Spread the strained pineapple evenly over the brown sugar. Arrange the cherries in two rows of 6 cherries each.

6. Gently pour the cake batter over the pineapples and cherries.

7. Place the baking dish on the grill and cook for 20 minutes. Rotate the baking dish 180 degrees and cook for 20 minutes more. The cake is done when a butter knife inserted into the center comes out clean.

8. Immediately run a knife around the inside of the baking dish to loosen the cake. Place a large serving platter or cutting board upside down onto the baking dish and turn over the platter and dish together. Gently pull the baking dish straight up, releasing the cake. Let the cake cool for at least 1 hour before serving.

BBQ EZ TIP: You can use 1 (15.25-ounce) box of yellow cake mix in place of the homemade cake mix, if you prefer. If using the boxed cake, skip step 3.

SMOKY BAKED APPLES

DIRECT HEAT COOKING
MAKES 6 APPLES ★ **PREP TIME:** 10 MINUTES ★ **COOK TIME:** 45 MINUTES
TOOLS: Apple or cherry wood chips, 9-by-13-inch baking dish

This baked apple recipe highlights fall's favorite fruit and accents it with a kiss of smoke. All you have to do is core the apples, fill them with buttery brown sugar, cinnamon, raisins, and nuts, then bake on the grill until slightly soft. For an added treat, serve with a scoop of vanilla bean ice cream.

- 6 Golden Delicious or Rome apples
- 6 tablespoons dark brown sugar
- 1½ teaspoons ground cinnamon
- 6 tablespoons raisins
- 6 tablespoons chopped walnuts (optional)
- 6 teaspoons cold unsalted butter, cut into 1-teaspoon slices
- ¾ cup boiling water
- Vanilla bean ice cream, for serving (optional)

1. Preheat the grill to medium heat (375°F) for direct heat cooking by lighting the heat source (or piling coals) in the spot that will be directly under the food. Add a handful of apple or cherry wood chips to the grill.

2. Rinse and dry the apples. Using a sharp paring knife or an apple corer, cut out the cores, leaving ½ inch of the bottom of the apple intact. Using a teaspoon, scoop out the seeds, leaving a 1-inch-wide hole through the middle of the apple.

3. In a small bowl, stir together the brown sugar, cinnamon, raisins, and walnuts (if using). Using a teaspoon, stuff the apples with the brown sugar mixture. Place a slice of butter on top of the sugar mixture in each apple.

4. Place the apples in a baking dish and pour the boiling water into the bottom of the dish, so it wets the bottoms of the apples.

5. Place the baking dish on the grill and cook the apples for 40 to 45 minutes, until they are cooked through and tender. When the apples are done, baste them with the juice from the baking dish.

6. Serve each apple with a scoop of vanilla ice cream (if using).

TRIPLE-BERRY CRISP

DIRECT HEAT COOKING
SERVES 8 ★ **PREP TIME:** 15 MINUTES ★ **COOK TIME:** 40 MINUTES
TOOLS: Cast-iron skillet, electric hand mixer

Our daughter Savanna loved to bake when she was little, and this was one of the very first things my wife and I taught her to make. This recipe is easy and packed with an assortment of mixed berries, which form a juicy filling nestled under a crisp and sugary topping.

- 2 pounds frozen mixed berries
- ¼ cup granulated sugar
- ⅓ cup freshly squeezed orange juice
- ⅔ cup all-purpose flour
- ¾ teaspoon baking powder
- ⅛ teaspoon kosher salt
- 8 tablespoons (1 stick) unsalted butter, melted
- ½ cup packed light brown sugar
- ½ teaspoon vanilla extract
- 1 large egg
- Whipped cream or whipped topping

1. Preheat the grill to medium heat (350°F) for direct heat cooking by lighting the heat source (or piling coals) in the spot that will be directly under the food.

2. In a medium bowl, stir together the berries, granulated sugar, and orange juice. Pour the berry mixture into a cast-iron skillet. In another medium bowl, whisk the flour, baking powder, and salt.

3. In another medium bowl, using an electric hand mixer, cream together the melted butter and brown sugar. Add the vanilla and egg and mix until fully incorporated. Slowly add the flour mixture and stir with a wooden spoon until incorporated but not overmixed.

4. Using a tablespoon, spoon the batter over the berries, dropping it in small clumps and leaving gaps between the batter, so the berries peek through.

5. Place the skillet on the grill and cook the crisp for 20 minutes. Rotate the skillet 180 degrees and cook for 20 minutes more. The crisp is done when the batter is golden brown and the berry mixture is bubbling. Remove the skillet from the grill and serve the hot crisp with whipped cream.

GRILLED CHERRY HAND PIES

DIRECT HEAT COOKING
SERVES 12 ★ PREP TIME: 15 MINUTES ★ **COOK TIME:** 15 MINUTES
TOOLS: Baking sheet, parchment paper, cherry wood chips (optional), 4-inch biscuit cutter

These little pockets of cherry grill up quickly in 15 minutes and make a great picnic treat that can easily be made ahead. I'm using cherry pie filling here, rather than fresh sour cherries, because they are hard to find and only available for a very short period of time each year. The cherry wood has a mild and fruity flavor and adds just the right amount of smoke flavor to this dish.

1 (14-ounce) package refrigerated (not frozen in the tin) piecrust (contains 2 piecrusts)

1 (21-ounce) can cherry pie filling

1 large egg white, beaten

2½ cups powdered sugar

1 teaspoon freshly squeezed lemon juice

¼ cup whole milk

1. Line a baking sheet with parchment paper.

2. Preheat the grill to medium-high heat (425°F) for direct heat cooking by lighting the heat source (or piling coals) in the spot that will be directly under the food. Add a handful of cherry wood chips to the grill (if using).

3. Unroll the piecrusts and use a 4-inch biscuit cutter to cut 6 circles from each crust, for a total of 12 circles (you may need to reroll the dough scraps to get the final circle from each crust).

4. Drop 1 tablespoon of cherry pie filling into the center of each piecrust circle. Fold the piecrust circles in half and pinch the edges closed completely. Press the edges with the tines of a fork to seal. Poke the hand pie once through the top only with the fork; the small holes will prevent the pie from bursting.

5. Place the hand pies on the prepared baking sheet about 1 inch apart. Brush the tops of the hand pies with the beaten egg white.

6. Place the baking sheet on the grill, close the lid, and cook the hand pies for 15 minutes, or until the crusts are golden brown.

7. In a medium bowl, whisk the powdered sugar, lemon juice, and milk until smooth.

8. Remove the hand pies from the grill, then carefully drop one hand pie into the icing mixture. Use two forks to remove it from the icing and return it to the parchment paper. Repeat with the remaining pies. Alternatively, put the icing in a zip-top bag, cut a hole in one of the corners, and drizzle the icing onto the hand pies. Let the icing set for 5 minutes before serving.

VARIATION TIP: This recipe is pretty universal and will work just about any pie filling. Some of my favorites are apple and strawberry. I avoid blackberry and raspberry fillings as they tend to have too many seeds.

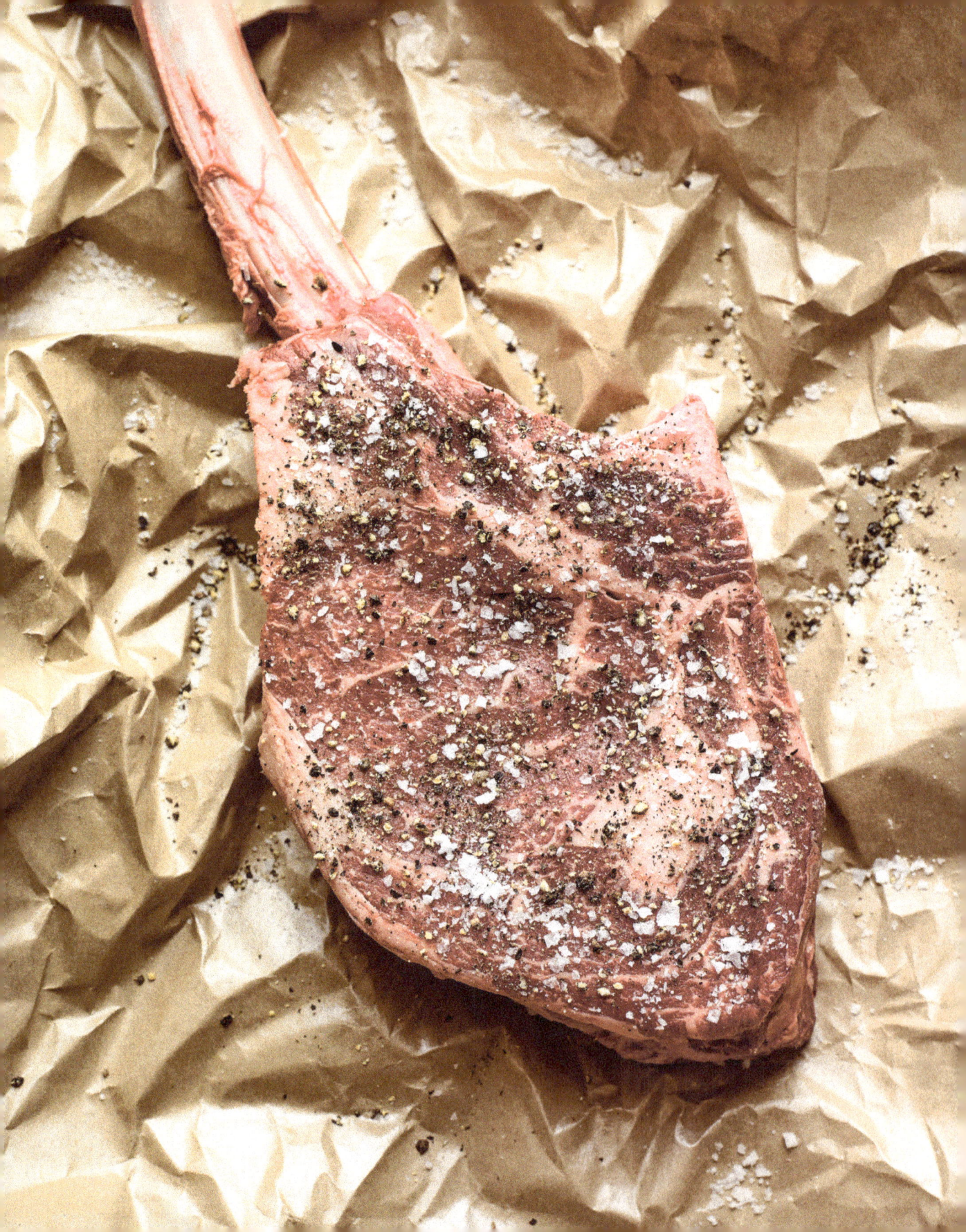

MEASUREMENT CONVERSIONS

VOLUME EQUIVALENTS	U.S. STANDARD	U.S. STANDARD (OUNCES)	METRIC (APPROXIMATE)
LIQUID	2 tablespoons	1 fl. oz.	30 mL
	¼ cup	2 fl. oz.	60 mL
	½ cup	4 fl. oz.	120 mL
	1 cup	8 fl. oz.	240 mL
	1½ cups	12 fl. oz.	355 mL
	2 cups or 1 pint	16 fl. oz.	475 mL
	4 cups or 1 quart	32 fl. oz.	1 L
	1 gallon	128 fl. oz.	4 L
DRY	⅛ teaspoon	—	0.5 mL
	¼ teaspoon	—	1 mL
	½ teaspoon	—	2 mL
	¾ teaspoon	—	4 mL
	1 teaspoon	—	5 mL
	1 tablespoon	—	15 mL
	¼ cup	—	59 mL
	⅓ cup	—	79 mL
	½ cup	—	118 mL
	⅔ cup	—	156 mL
	¾ cup	—	177 mL
	1 cup	—	235 mL
	2 cups or 1 pint	—	475 mL
	3 cups	—	700 mL
	4 cups or 1 quart	—	1 L
	½ gallon	—	2 L
	1 gallon	—	4 L

OVEN TEMPERATURES

FAHRENHEIT	CELSIUS (APPROXIMATE)
250°F	120°C
300°F	150°C
325°F	165°C
350°F	180°C
375°F	190°C
400°F	200°C
425°F	220°C
450°F	230°C

WEIGHT EQUIVALENTS

U.S. STANDARD	METRIC (APPROXIMATE)
½ ounce	15 g
1 ounce	30 g
2 ounces	60 g
4 ounces	115 g
8 ounces	225 g
12 ounces	340 g
16 ounces or 1 pound	455 g

INDEX

A
Appetizers cheat sheet, 18
Apples, Smoky Baked, 112
Applesauce, Maple-Bourbon Pork Chops with Smoked, 44–45
Asparagus, Pancetta-Wrapped, 102

B
Bacon
   Bacon Smash Burgers, 30–31
   Bacon-Wrapped Jalapeño Poppers, 19
   Moink Balls, 22
BBQ rub, 5
BBQ sauce, Kansas City–Style, 5
Beef
   Bacon Smash Burgers, 30–31
   Beef Short Ribs, 35
   cheat sheet, 28–29
   Cheesy Meat Loaf "Parmesan," 32–33
   Grilled Beef Fajita Salad with Cilantro-Lime Dressing, 36–37
   Grilled Santa Maria–Style Tri-Tip, 34
   Moink Balls, 22
   Reverse Seared Cowboy Steak with Chimichurri Sauce, 38–39
Berry Crisp, Triple-, 113
Black pepper, 3
Blueberry and Peach Galette, 108
Brown sugar, 4
Burgers, Bacon Smash, 30–31

C
Canola oil, 4
Carrots, Honey-Bourbon, 90
Cauliflower Mac and Cheese, Grilled, 88–89
Cedar Plank Teriyaki Salmon, 81
Charcoal grills
   charcoal vs. briquettes, 10
   lighting, 9–10
   smoking on, 14
Cheese
   Cheesy Meat Loaf "Parmesan," 32–33
   Green Chile–Cheese Corn Bread, 91
   Grilled Cauliflower Mac and Cheese, 88–89
   Jalapeño-Cheese Skillet Dip, 21
   Parmesan-Crusted Grilled Whitefish, 79
   Smoked Funeral Potatoes, 97
   Stuffed Poblano Peppers, 98–99
Cherry Hand Pies, Grilled, 114–115
Chicken
   Charcoal Chimney Yakitori Chicken, 66–67
   cheat sheet, 50–51
   Citrus-Marinated Chicken, 54
   Grilled Chicken Tinga, 55
   Grilled Huli Huli–Style Chicken, 57
   Grilled Nashville Hot Chicken, 61
   Lemon-Dijon-Rosemary Skewers, 58–59
   Maple-Dijon Grilled Chicken, 60
   Pollo al Carbon, 62–63
   Spicy Korean-Style Chicken, 52–53
Chimichurri Sauce, Reverse Seared Cowboy Steak with, 38–39
Chipotle chiles, 6
Cilantro-Lime Dressing, Grilled Beef Fajita Salad with, 36–37

Citrus-Marinated Chicken, 54
Corn
  Foil Packet Shrimp "Boil," 73
  Green Chile–Cheese Corn Bread, 91
  Grilled Mexican Street Corn (Elotes), 93
Cumin, 5

D

Desserts
  Blueberry and Peach Galette, 108
  cheat sheet, 106–107
  Grilled Cherry Hand Pies, 114–115
  Grilled S'mores Dip, 109
  Pineapple Upside-Down Cake, 110–111
  Smoky Baked Apples, 112
  Triple-Berry Crisp, 113
Direct fire, 11

E

Eggs, Smoked Deviled, 24–25

F

Fish and seafood
  Cajun Blackened Grilled Fish, 74–75
  Cedar Plank Teriyaki Salmon, 81
  cheat sheet, 70–71
  Foil Packet Shrimp "Boil," 73
  Grilled Swordfish with Red Pepper Sauce, 76–77
  Jamaican Jerk Grilled Halibut, 78
  Parmesan-Crusted Grilled Whitefish, 79
  Sweet Chili Shrimp, 72
  Tilapia Puttanesca, 82
Fry Sauce, Grilled Sweet Potatoes with, 94–95

G

Garlic, granulated, 4
Gas grills
  gas gauge hack, 10
  lighting, 9
  smoking on, 15
Green Chile–Cheese Corn Bread, 91
Grills
  cleaning, 13
  lighting, 9–10
  smoking on, 14–15

H

Halibut, Jamaican Jerk Grilled, 78
Honey-Bourbon Carrots, 90

I

Indirect fire, 11

J

Jalapeño peppers
  Bacon-Wrapped Jalapeño Poppers, 19
  Fire-Roasted Salsa, 20
  Jalapeño-Cheese Skillet Dip, 21

L

Lemon-Dijon-Rosemary Skewers, 58–59
Lime juice, 5
Liquid smoke, 6

M

Maple-Bourbon Pork Chops with Smoked Applesauce, 44–45
Maple-Dijon Grilled Chicken, 60
Mise en place, 2
Moink Balls, 22

O

Onion, granulated, 4

P

Pancetta-Wrapped Asparagus, 102
Paprika, 6
Parmesan-Crusted Grilled Whitefish, 79
Peach Galette, Blueberry and, 108
Pineapple Upside-Down Cake, 110–111
Poblano Peppers, Stuffed, 98–99

Pork. *See also* Bacon; Sausage
  Char Siu Pork Tenderloin, 46–47
  cheat sheet, 28–29
  Cheesy Meat Loaf "Parmesan," 32–33
  Grilled Al Pastor Skewers, 42–43
  Korean-Style Short Ribs, 41
  Maple-Bourbon Pork Chops with Smoked Applesauce, 44–45
Potatoes
  Foil Packet Shrimp "Boil," 73
  Poppa Joe's Camp Potatoes, 96
  Smoked Funeral Potatoes, 97
  Twice-Cooked Planked Potatoes, 100–101

R

Red Pepper Sauce, Grilled Swordfish with, 76–77

S

Salmon, Cedar Plank Teriyaki, 81
Salsa, Fire-Roasted, 20
Salt, 3, 6
Sausage
  Cheesy Meat Loaf "Parmesan," 32–33
  Foil Packet Shrimp "Boil," 73
Seafood. *See* Fish and seafood
Shrimp
  Foil Packet Shrimp "Boil," 73
  Sweet Chili Shrimp, 72

Skewers
  Grilled Al Pastor Skewers, 42–43
  Lemon-Dijon-Rosemary Skewers, 58–59
Smoke flavorings, 6
Smoking foods, 13–15
S'mores Dip, Grilled, 109
Sweet Chili Shrimp, 72
Sweet Potatoes with Fry Sauce, Grilled, 94–95
Swordfish with Red Pepper Sauce, Grilled, 76–77

T

Temperature ranges, 12
Tilapia Puttanesca, 82
Tools and equipment, 7–8
Turbinado sugar, 4
Turkey
  Central Texas–Style BBQ Turkey Breast, 64–65
  cheat sheet, 50–51
Two-zone indirect fire, 11

V

Vegetables cheat sheet, 86–87
Vinegar, 4

W

Watermelon Wedges, Grilled, 23
Wood chips and pellets, 14

ACKNOWLEDGMENTS

Thanks to my wife, Vida, for her extraordinary patience, understanding, and support while I was maintaining a crazy schedule to complete this book. Thanks for believing in me! Special thanks to David Nelson and the team at Crawford Outdoors for the use of their Napoleon Prestige Pro 500 grill for the development of these tasty recipes. This book would not have been possible without the support of the Callisto Media/Rockridge Press team, especially Georgia Freedman, my editor, who guided me along this journey.

ABOUT THE AUTHOR

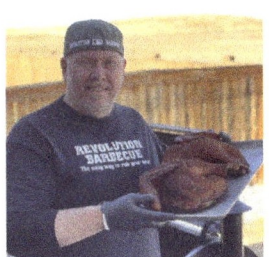

Glenn Connaughton is the creator of the Revolution Barbecue brand. After years of competing on the barbecue competition circuit and running a catering business, Glenn has turned his focus to growing the brand and sharing his love of barbecue on social media. When not commanding the grill, you can find Glenn enjoying the outdoors with his wife, Vida, and his adult children in Colorado. Find him @revolutionbbq.

www.ingramcontent.com/pod-product-compliance
Lightning Source LLC
LaVergne TN
LVHW070948070426
835507LV00029B/3458